Medical Questions Answered
What You Always Wanted to Ask Your Doctor

Medical Questions Answered

What You Always Wanted to Ask Your Doctor

Ray M. Schilling, MD

Medical Questions Answered
What You Always Wanted to Ask Your Doctor
Ray M. Schilling, MD

Copyright © 2018 by Ray M. Schilling, MD
All Rights Reserved

Book and Cover Design by Karoline Butler

ISBN-10: 1986276015
ISBN-13: 978-1986276016
Library of Congress Control Number: 2018939075

Published by KKCalifornia
Palm Desert, California

Acknowledgments

I like to thank my wife, Christina Schilling for proof-reading this book and giving me valuable input with regard to the illustrations. I also like to thank Karoline Butler for helping with the cover design, the interior (layout, design, images etc.) and helping with the publication process.

Dedication

I dedicate this book to you, the reader. I am fully aware that you may have some of the diseases and conditions that I described and answered in this book. I wish you a speedy recovery from any health problem that you are experiencing. Also I like to recommend to you to become more proactive and put emphasis on prevention, as I pointed out in many of the questions I answered.

Contents

My Background xvii

About this Book xxi

1: Acne 1
What is the best home remedy for acne (pimples)?

2: Aging 9
What are some of the surprising facts about aging?
What unexpected things occur when you age?
Why does Bill Gate's face look relatively old?
Can aging be reversed in the future?
Can aging be reversed?
Why is immortality impossible?
Is it impossible to extend the human lifespan?
Anti-aging: what are some of the best tips?
What limits the age for a human?
What is life like in your 70's?

3: Alcohol 31
How does alcohol affect your body?
Does beer change your body temperature?

4: Alzheimer's Disease 33
Could it be that sugar overconsumption causes Alzheimer's disease?
Why do people experience memory decline?
Which foods promote brain health?
What are the latest suggested causes of Alzheimer's disease?

5: Appearance 46
Why do some people have chin dimples?

6: Arthritis 47
What can cause rheumatoid arthritis and how do you treat it?
What can you do about osteoarthritis?
How does gout develop?

7: Autism 53
Is it true that vaccines cause autism?

8: Back Pain 55
Treating symptoms of back pain only is insufficient
Running on a treadmill I get lower back pain. What should I do?
When I am angry, I tend to get lower back pain. Why is this?

9: Brain 58
What is the dark part about the brain?

10: Cancer 60
Could the increased consumption of processed food in the past 50 years be responsible for a rise in cancer?
Does smoking a few cigarettes cause lung cancer?

Is smoking cigarettes really causing cancer?
Is cancer caused by a lack of exercise and wrong food choices?
Can cancer ever be turned into a disease we can live with?
Can cancer cells metabolize more glucose than normal cells?
Could you get cancer from makeup?
I have a lump in the esophagus; I find it progressively more difficult to swallow. Must I seek the advice of a physician, when I know that esophagus cancer cannot be treated?
Is there a method that will only kill cancer cells, but not normal cells?
If old age or disease won't kill you, will cancer do it?
Can cinnamon and coffee be used in the fight against cancer?
Why are cancer cells so difficult to identify; are there no cell markers that would give them away in at test?
Why can cancer still not be cured? When will this change?
Cancer is difficult to treat, is it a supernatural disease?
Is there a "sour honey cure" of cancer?
Is it true that oncologists, if they come down with cancer themselves will refuse chemotherapy?
Warning signs for cancer

11: Contraception 88
Can she get pregnant, if he pulled it out, cleaned it and reinserted it again?
Can I get pregnant, if he just inserts his penis?
How does a married couple avoid pregnancy when they have sex?

12: Death 90
Why do people die of old age?

13: Depression 92
Will my depression ever go away? I have tried drugs and exercise, but nothing seems to work. Sometimes I am suicidal.

14: Detoxification **103**
Does the skin help in detoxifying the body?

15: Diabetes **104**
Will a 600 Calorie diet help diabetes control?
Is chicken and mutton OK to eat for diabetics?

16: Diet **106**
Anti-inflammatory diet: Mediterranean diet
I want to get rid of sugar in my diet. How can I do this long-term?
What would happen, if I removed all sugar except fruit and honey from my diet?
Is there one particular food component that makes us fat and obese?
Can you live for 4 years on only microwave cooked food?
Why do dieticians often support nutritional principles that are miles apart, for instance Vegan versus Paleo versus Mediterranean diets?
I have poor eating habits and also bad sleeping habits. Does that affect my health?
Why do some Americans prefer processed, preserved or packaged foods to farm-fresh food?
Are fruit unhealthy due to their sugar content?
Is there a difference between cheap and expensive chocolate?
Some foods are advertised healthy, but they are actually not?
What is the difference between regular and steel-cut oats?
Too much refined sugar can make you sick. Is it as bad as cigarettes?
Let's assume I don't eat sugar for one year. What would happen?
What are some key facts about healthy food consumption?
Thought experiment: take our food from today and introduce it into a medieval village in Europe. What would happen to the population?

I have eaten a lot of unhealthy food. What's the best thing I can do to become healthier now?
Is mouldy bread bad for me? Should I microwave it?
Xylitol against tooth decay
Consequences of a one-week fast
Is there are difference between Irish butter and American butter?

17: Digestion **138**
Can you develop an ulcer in your stomach from not eating regularly?
I am passing a lot of gas. What could be the cause?
If I bring up yellow vomit, what does it mean?

18: Doctor **148**
As a doctor, have you diagnosed yourself and averted an emergency?
What stands out in your career as a doctor as a most memorable moment?
Do you get compensated for a call: "Is there a doctor on the flight?"

19: Exercise **152**
How useful is cardiovascular exercise?
Does running or any other exercise help you to lose weight?
Could running marathons be dangerous for you?

20: Fate **155**
What did you find sad about your mother and/or father?

21: Foot Problems **157**
What is plantar fasciitis and how do you treat it?

22: Gut Disease **159**
Is "gluten free" food healthy?

23: Heart 162
Could we replace the heart with an artificial pump and live forever?

24: Heart Disease 164
What can I do to clean out my arteries and reduce my risk for heart disease?
How do you assess the risk for heart disease in the elderly?
Are statins required by anybody with high cholesterol?

25: High Blood Pressure 179
Are there treatments other than drugs to treat high blood pressure?
Is the wall of the left heart chamber always thicker than the right one?

26: Hormones 183
Is estrogen present in the male body?
Is testosterone effective?
Why does testosterone production in a male decrease with age?
How can I increase testosterone and lower estrogen in my blood?
I was diagnosed with hypothyroidism and started on levothyroxine. How long before I will be better?
Does flaxseed consumption decrease testosterone levels?
What is unexpected when you get old?

27: Hospital 195
Why do physicians keep some patients in hospital overnight?

28: Infections 197
Can you turn blind from sharing your bed with your cat?
Why do I have a sore throat?

29: Injuries 200
Ear drum injury by Q-tip
How dangerous is it to bite your tongue?

30: Keeping Your Brain Healthy 203
Foods for brain health

31: Life Expectancy 206
What is the theoretical life expectancy of humans?
What is the life expectancy for humans in this day and age?
Do exercise and diet influence your life expectancy?
Health impact of smoking cigarettes and drinking alcohol
How come it is impossible to extend the human lifespan beyond a certain limit?

32: Lifestyle Habits 214
Can good habits change your life completely?
How did key happenings in your life change your life direction?
What things do I need to do every day to get the best out of life?
Can smoking and drinking ruin my health?

33: Pain 225
Pain relief for a headache or other pain: Aleve, Advil or Tylenol?

34: Parenting 228
Has the old slogan "tough love" backfired?

35: Pregnancy 229
I am pregnant and following my first ultrasound scan I was told that my baby is not healthy. I was advised abort. What should I do?
How can a female get pregnant?
Best age for successful pregnancy

36: Prostate Cancer 231
How dangerous is prostate cancer? Does it kill you?

37: Schizophrenia 235
What complementary approach may help a patient with schizophrenia?

38: Skin 238
Can I apply Aloe Vera gel on my face overnight?

39: Sleep 239
What time does it take to fall asleep?
What you need to know about sleep
What happens when you go to bed late every night?
Is going to bed at 5 AM and waking up at 1 PM unhealthy?
Will a drug ever be developed that eliminates the need for sleep?
Could genetic engineering help humans one day to only need 1 or 2 hours of sleep daily?
How much would the average person gain from one hour of extra sleep?
What are the nuts and bolts about sleeping?
I sleep from midnight until 7:30 AM, but I am extremely groggy in the morning. Why?
I have to work night shifts (9 PM to 6:30 AM). How will this affect my health?
Why do we have to sleep 7-8 hours a night, why not just 4 hours?
If I sleep for 6 hours, am I getting enough sleep?

40: Sugar 257
Will I be OK living without sugar?
Effects of sugar on our health
If I cut out sugar, what will happen?

41: Vaccinations 261
Is there a connection between vaccinations and autism?

42: Vitamins and Supplements 263
Are taking vitamins and supplements healthy or are they harmful?
The all-important vitamin D
Why does turmeric fight cancer?

43: Weight Loss 283
I am working out every day, but I am not loosing weight. What should I do?
I lost weight on a diet, but now I am afraid of regaining weight, if I eat normally. Can you tell me what to do?
How can I get rid of belly fat, and then maintain a good-looking body?
My stomach is outgrowing my pants. Would 30 minutes jogging a day help?
How can I lose weight without too much exercise?
Can I get a flat belly by just running every day without crunches?
How can I get rid of my lower belly fat?

44: Younger for Longer 291
Why are some people younger looking than their stated age?
When do we develop wrinkles in our face?
What are three things I can do every day to stay younger for longer?

45: Summary 297

Index 299

My Background

I studied medicine in a traditional medical school in Germany (Tübingen University). After a rotating internship at Tübingen University teaching hospitals I moved to Canada.

My working career can be described in three sections.

- First, I spent a bit more than 3 years in cancer research at the Ontario Cancer Institute, located at the Princess Margaret Hospital, Toronto, ON. It has since been renamed "The Princess Margaret Cancer Centre".
- Secondly, after 2 ½ years of more training at McMaster University, Hamilton, ON, and passing the Canadian State examination (the LMCC exam) I practiced medicine in my own family medicine practice for 16 years in a suburb of Vancouver, BC in Southern British Columbia.
- Finally, from 1994 until my retirement in 2010 I was a medical advisor for WorkSafeBC solving occupational medicine problems.

In all three phases of my career I was required to answer medical questions. In cancer research experiments were conducted to see what was required to mount an immune response to cancer cells. The findings were published in medical papers. My fellow researchers and I were challenged by difficult questions with regard to the biology of cancer development that we tried to answer.

In general practice it was the patients that I treated, and they wanted to get answers to medical questions. Why did they develop pneumonia? They always had been healthy. So, why would they come down with cancer now? I answered their questions as best as I could.

After my switch to occupational medicine the questions were different. The case managers wanted to know whether the findings as reported by a specialist would be due to a work-related injury or whether they were due to a pre-existing condition. Work-related injuries were considered part of the Workers' Compensation claim, but pre-existing conditions were not covered under the claim.

When you keep on answering medical questions for 35 years it becomes second nature of you to do this. It is with this background that I had the idea that I should write this book.

Ray M. Schilling, MD
Kelowna, BC, Canada
May 2018

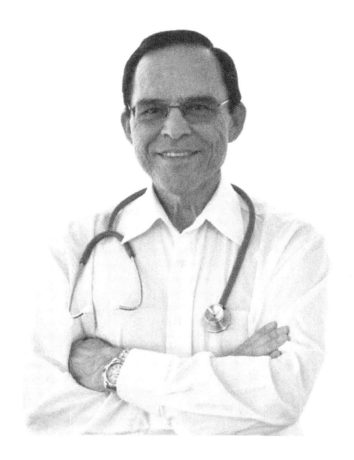

Ray M. Schilling, MD - 2018

About This Book

1. You may be missing individual chapters in this book. Instead I have arranged more than 120 medical questions under more than 40 headings. To make it simpler for the reader, the headings are listed in the beginning of the book alphabetically. Under each heading you find one or more questions that belong to this topic. The same order is kept in the book (questions arranged under alphabetical headings). For those of you who would prefer to look up a subject in an index I have also added an exhaustive index at the end of the book.
2. You may wonder why I chose these particular questions in this book. I was guided by popularity of questions over a long period of time. People want to know about sleep patterns, diets, cancer cures, heart disease, exercise, and aging, back pain, arthritis, Alzheimer's disease and more. All of these headings are included and you find many answers to these topics.
3. You may also wonder why I answered some questions with only a few paragraphs, but others with a much longer answer. With some questions I felt a short answer would suffice. With other answers I felt that I

should give some broad background information first and only then answer these questions.

4. The key in the book is that in all answers to questions I am attempting to point out the importance of being proactive. This is particularly important with early cancer detection and treatment. But any other disease should be diagnosed as early as possible and treated before it becomes an emergency. A lot of suffering can be prevented this way, and long-term outlooks are much better.

I am hoping that you get as much from the answered questions as I intended to give to you. I have provided many links to other web sites that will also provide you with more information regarding the question. But I encourage you to ask more questions from your health provider and also research the Internet. There are so many good health web sites that you can consult.

All of this will broaden your knowledge. And this leads to making better decisions! Being an informed consumer helps you to take better care of your health, ask the right questions and get better care.

Every effort was taken that all website links quoted in this book were functioning properly at the time of publishing. However, due to updates or changes they may result in outdated links.

Disclaimer

This book will help you to consider treatment options for many health conditions. If you want to apply any of these in your own healthcare, discuss it with your physician or alternative healthcare provider. The legal responsibility remains with you and your healthcare provider. This book is not an "instruction manual for self treatment", but it is geared to turning you into an "informed consumer" To your health!

Chapter 1:

Acne

What is the best home remedy for acne (pimples)?

    Who would have thought that acne could come from a combination of sugar and milk products? Careful epidemiological studies have shown that in some regions of Africa, Brazil and Japan teenagers who eat the local food do not get acne, but when they switch to a Western style diet they come down with acne.
    There has been a renewed interest in the last 40 years to sort out the connection between dietary factors and acne (1).
    It appears from the studies below that the cause of acne is poor nutrition, so it makes sense to use a nutritional approach first to treat acne.
The most straightforward treatment in my opinion is to modify what you eat.
    A clinical trial from the University of Melbourne in 2007 showed that a low-glycemic diet reduced the acne lesions by 22% compared to a control group (2).
    Two factors are clear: a low-glycemic diet produces fewer pimples, the stricter a low-glycemic diet is applied, the more effective the treatment will be. Up to 50% reduction in acne lesions were observed among patients with acne who adhered to a strict low-glycemic index diet in just 12

weeks. There is also evidence that milk and other dairy products can contribute to acne, which works through the same mechanism of IGF-1 stimulation mentioned above (3).

A US study from Boston showed a 22% increase in acne lesions with total milk consumption and increase of 44% after skim milk consumption (4).

Omega-3-fatty acid supplementation is useful for inflammatory acne in about 2/3 of the cases as this study showed (5).

Here is a patient from this study who benefitted from omega-3 supplementation.

The baseline image is seen with inflammatory acne lesions on his cheek (6).

Only 12 weeks after taking 3 Grams of omega-3 supplementation daily his face looked much improved (7).

Facts about acne

For a long time nobody knew why teenagers get acne. But many assumed that it would come from hormonal changes as teenagers grow up. But why then are there some ethnic regions in the world where teenagers do not get acne? In this blog I will present the background that shows that wheat, sugar and dairy products are the culprits. They are not eaten in those regions of our planet where acne does not exist.

Regions where acne does not exist

1. The Kitivan Islanders of Papua New Guinea have no cases of acne in teenagers (8). They adhere to the old hunter/gatherer diet of no sugar, no alcohol, no wheat and no grains (9). Instead they eat root vegetables such as sweet potato, yam, taro, tapioca; fruit like papaya, pineapple, banana, mango, watermelon, guava and pumpkin; and also vegetables, coconuts and fish.

2. African Bantus and Zulus: These original African warriors eat a low glycemic diet with no wheat, no milk and no refined sugar or starches (10). Their teenagers and young adult do not have acne, if they stick to the original tribal diet.

3. Aché hunter/gatherers of Paraguay: a study by researchers from the Colorado State University in 2002 showed that sugar, wheat and other high-glycemic foods were missing in the diet of these native tribes. As a result they have no acne when they consume this type of diet, which is very similar to the Kitivan Islanders of Papua New Guinea.

4. Japan's Okinawans, when sticking to their original diet before 1970, had a clear complexion and no pimples (acne). But as this link shows the McDonald's and other fast foods with too much salt, too much sugar, wheat, deep fried and convenience foods entered the scene after 1970 and the acne rate went up to the American level.

5. The natives of the Purus Valley in Brazil: A dermatological examination of 9955 school children age 6 to 16 showed an acne incidence of only 2.7% (11). In contrast in Westernized countries the rate of acne is 60 to 80%. The diet in this region is again similar to the other groups already mentioned above.

6. Canadian Inuit before 1950 did not consume dairy products and were acne free (12). Since then there has been a steady increase of dairy products, soda, beef, and processed foods.

How acne develops

The medical term for pimples or acne is "acne vulgaris". For years it has been postulated that hormones and medication can cause acne (13).

According to Rakel there are several steps that work together in causing acne. The hair follicle and sebaceous gland work as one unit. Male hormones, called androgens play an important role in the development of acne, both in males and females. Testosterone in males is not only produced in testicles, but also in the skin itself. It gets converted by an enzyme, 5-alpha-reductase, into the much more active metabolite dihydrotestosterone. In individuals with hypersensitive receptors in the sebaceous gland this will cause blockage in the sebaceous gland duct and at the same time stimulate the sebaceous gland oil production leading to the formation of a keratotic plug. White heads and black heads are formed this way (14).

Contributing factors are inflammatory substances that are caused by insulin release stimulated by sugar, wheat and starch intake. This stimulates IGF-1 receptors in the skin, which causes growth of the subcutaneous skin layers, which is pushing up from the layer below the skin, kinking the sebaceous gland duct and causing acne pustules (pimples) to form. A skin bacterium, called Propionibacterium acnes (P. acnes), is getting trapped in the pimple causing a local skin infection, which in turn can cause acne cysts and furuncles, particularly in males where there is a family history of acne. High cortisol levels from stress can also be a contributing factor in causing acne. Today's teenagers are exposed to a lot of stresses from exams, competitive sports and peer pressure.

Females with PCOS (polycystic ovary syndrome) have higher androgen production from ovarian cysts, which results in acne as well.

Both male and female teenagers experience an androgen surge when puberty sets in. If the teenager avoids the additional insulin response, which comes from eating sugar, starch, grain and particularly from consuming wheat and wheat products, the plugging up of skin pores will not occur, meaning these teenagers will be acne free. Some teenagers are also sensitive to milk protein from milk and milk products. In sensitive people whey protein allergy causes the same insulin/skin IGF-1 response described above, which leads to blocking of skin pores. If there is no blockage in the hair follicle, the P. acnes bacteria will stay on the surface of the skin (these bacteria are part of the normal skin flora) and the sebaceous gland secretions flow unimpededly to the surface of the skin keeping it naturally lubricated. These observations are further confirmed by a study from Malaysia in 2012 showing that a high glycemic load diet with milk and ice cream caused worsening of acne in teenagers of both sexes (15).

Treating acne correctly

A) Conventional acne treatment

This is a thorny issue, because Big Pharma has a firm hand in the treatment of acne and they are supporting symptomatic treatment of acne rather than treating the cause. There are surface treatment modalities that are supposed to open the skin pores: peeling agents such as benzoyl peroxide. General practitioners often treat the infection with antibiotic pills (tetracycline or erythromycin), but this is not treating the cause, only the super infection that comes from the plugged up skin pores (stasis of sebaceous gland secretions). Another approach is topical application of antibiotic and peeling agent in combination (1% clindamycin and 5% benzoyl peroxide gel), which is applied twice daily (Mandell et al.). Resistant cases, usually the ones who have a family history of severe acne, have been treated by a skin specialist who has a special license to treat with isotretinoin (Accutane), a vitamin A derivative, which works in many cases, but which can have serious side effects (16).
These include skin dryness, eye dryness, muscle and bone pains, headaches, liver enzyme abnormalities, and

instability of mood including depression and causing birth defects in the fetus of a pregnant woman (Cleveland Clinic). In 2009 the manufacturer stopped distributing the drug in the US, because of too many lawsuits regarding damages from the drug.

I am not saying you should ever take this toxic medication. What I am saying is that treating symptoms, but not the cause has led to peculiar drug manufacturing. This drug is now used to treat brain cancer and pancreatic cancer.

B) Dietary approach to treat acne

There has been a renewed interest in the last 40 years to sort out the connection between dietary factors and acne (17).

The most straightforward treatment in my opinion is to modify what you eat.

A clinical trial from the University of Melbourne in 2007 showed that a low-glycemic diet reduced the acne lesions by 22% compared to a control group (18).

Two factors are clear: a low-glycemic diet produces fewer pimples, the stricter the low-glycemic diet is applied, the more effective the treatment will be. Up to 50% reduction in acne lesions were observed among patients with acne who adhered to a strict low-glycemic index diet in just 12 weeks. There is also evidence that milk and other dairy products can contribute to acne, which works through the same mechanism of IGF-1 stimulation mentioned above (19).

A US study from Boston showed a 22% increase in acne lesions with total milk consumption and increase of 44% after skim milk consumption (20).

Conclusion

There is a lesson to be learnt from the analysis of the regions in the world where acne does not exist and from all these observational studies mentioned. Cutting out wheat, wheat products, grains, sugar, milk and milk products will lead to amazing results regarding acne prevention and improvement of patients who suffer from acne. We have been lulled into believing that medical science will give us a magic pill or magic potion that would solve our complexion problems. As mentioned above one of the "magic pills" (isotretinoin) is so toxic that it is now used for cancer treatments. All along we allowed the food industry to destroy our complexion by inducing an insulin and IGF-1 response that plugged up our skin pores. We can open them up by eliminating wheat and wheat products, sugar, high-glycemic foods as well as dairy products.

More information on acne: http://nethealthbook.com/dermatology-skin-disease/acne-vulgaris/

Book references

1. Rakel: Integrative Medicine, 3rd ed., Saunders 2012. Chapter 73 : Acne Vulgaris and Acne Rosacea, by Sean H. Zager, MD
2. Mandell, Douglas, and Bennett's Principles and Practice of Infectious Diseases, 7th ed., © 2009 Churchill Livingstone.
3. Cleveland Clinic: Current Clinical Medicine, 2nd ed., © 2010 Saunders.

Note: This blog was previously published here: http://www.askdrray.com/pimples-and-acne-can-be-caused-by-food/

Internet references

1. https://www.ncbi.nlm.nih.gov/pubmed/23438493
2. https://www.ncbi.nlm.nih.gov/pubmed/17448569
3. https://www.ncbi.nlm.nih.gov/pubmed/19709092

4. https://www.ncbi.nlm.nih.gov/pubmed/15692464
5. https://www.ncbi.nlm.nih.gov/pubmed/23206895
6. https://www.ncbi.nlm.nih.gov/pmc/articles/PMC3543297/figure/F3/
7. https://www.ncbi.nlm.nih.gov/pmc/articles/PMC3543297/figure/F4/
8. https://www.ncbi.nlm.nih.gov/pubmed/12472346
9. http://www.paleoplan.com/2011/05-18/hunter-gatherer-profile-the-kitavans/
10. https://risefigure.wordpress.com/health-archive/acne/acne-preventing-acne/
11. https://www.ncbi.nlm.nih.gov/pubmed/7274519
12. https://en.wikipedia.org/wiki/Inuit_cuisine
13. https://www.ncbi.nlm.nih.gov/pubmed/19932324
14. https://herbalorganic.wordpress.com/whiteheads-and-blackheads/
15. https://bmcdermatol.biomedcentral.com/articles/10.1186/1471-5945-12-13
16. https://en.wikipedia.org/wiki/Isotretinoin
17. https://www.ncbi.nlm.nih.gov/pubmed/23438493
18. https://www.ncbi.nlm.nih.gov/pubmed/17448569
19. https://www.ncbi.nlm.nih.gov/pubmed/19709092
20. https://www.ncbi.nlm.nih.gov/pubmed/15692464

Chapter 2:

Aging

What are some of the surprising facts about aging?

1. Until not too long ago scientists thought that aging was a one-way street. Your DNA ages, mitochondria, the cells' power plants age and the telomeres get shorter as we age. At the end we run out of steam and die. In one study the telomere length at the age of 100 was only 40% of the average length of telomeres of the group at the age of 20.

2. Now we are learning that telomeres can be lengthened by healthy lifestyles. It has been shown in humans that increased physical activity elongated telomeres. So did vitamin C, E and vitamin D3 supplementation, resveratrol, a Mediterranean diet and marine omega-3 fatty acid supplementation. In addition higher fiber intake, bioidentical estrogen in women and testosterone in men, relaxation techniques like yoga and meditation are also elongating telomeres.

3. Mitochondria can be preserved through exercise, CoQ-10 supplementation and caloric restriction (1).

4. Another factor of aging is hormone deficiency in general and growth hormone (GH) deficiency in particular.

Here is a review article about human growth hormone deficiency that may be mind-blowing to you (2).

When people age, they lose GH production, which puts them at a considerable risk to get heart attacks and strokes, but they are also at a higher risk of serious falls due to muscle weakness and balance problems. When the doctor detects low IGF-1 levels in the blood and confirms low GH metabolites in a 24-hour urine sample, the time has come to do daily GH injections with human GH. This can be done using a similar pen that is used for insulin injections. The dosage is very small- only between 0.1 mg and 0.2 mg per day, given before bedtime. This is remarkably effective not only for heart attack and stroke prevention, but also to treat muscle weakness, lack of mental clarity and to preserve general well being. Patients report that their joint and muscle aches disappear, and they can engage in physical activities again. But GH is not the only hormone that needs to be observed and possibly be replaced by nature-identical hormones (3).

Conclusion

We have the tools nowadays to postpone aging considerably. The key is to approach this scientifically; think about your mitochondria (where energy comes from), your telomeres, because you need healthy DNA; your hormones, good nutrition and exercise. This provides a healthy framework on which you can build healthy aging.

Internet references

1. https://www.drwhitaker.com/3-ways-to-tune-up-your-mitochondria-and-enhance-energy/
2. https://www.ncbi.nlm.nih.gov/pmc/articles/PMC3183535/
3. http://www.askdrray.com/effects-of-hormones-on-the-heart/

What unexpected things occur when you age?

Hormone deficiencies are what many people do not expect.

1. You get muscle aches and pains, and your energy is missing. Your sleep is getting shallower and you wake up several times during the night. Your doctor suspects that you may have a hormonal problem. Your thyroid-stimulating hormone (TSH) is 14.6 and your T3 and T4 hormones are low. After some thyroid hormones (Armour, which is a mix of T3 and T4) your energy comes back, your muscle aches and pains disappear and you sleep again the way you used to do it.

2. Any man most likely likes to have his regular sex life. It can happen as early as in the fifties that there is a problem in this department. Erections are not what they used to be and he finds it more difficult to reach orgasm. Instead of every 2 days, he only wants sex every 3 to 4 days. He sees his family doctor and a testosterone level test will be ordered. A low level of testosterone shows up on a blood test. The doctor starts him on twice weekly testosterone self-injections. Within 2 weeks his regular sex life returns, quite to the astonishment of him and to the delight of his wife.

3. Back to sleep problems. Some people have problems in their 30's or 40's to fall asleep. Melatonin is the known hormone from the pineal gland that initiates and maintains sleep. Melatonin happens to be the human hormone that vanishes first with aging. Already above the age of 20 to 30 melatonin production begins to decline. It's clear, why many people benefit from a 3 mg dose of melatonin at bedtime. This could be repeated should you wake up in the middle of the night. There is no side effect, because melatonin is a hormone that the body knows.

4. Menopause and andropause also affect hormone production. We've already discussed the lack of testosterone in andropause. But women also need hormone replacement when they enter menopause.

Conclusion

Many people are surprised by the decline in hormone production, as one gets older. They should supplement with bioidentical hormones to rebalance the hormone system.

Why does Bill Gate's face look relatively old?

Aging is a complex topic. There are many factors that cause premature aging. One big factor is being exposed to too much stress, which means your cortisol level is high. Cortisol can shorten telomeres, the caps at the end of chromosomes, which ages you prematurely.

We lose hair pigment with aging, but a bit of hair color could give you a younger look, if the grey bothers you!

Wrinkles come from a lack of human growth hormone (HGH), which gives you an older appearance. As we age, we produce less HGH (see my answer to this question under Life expectancy: What is the life expectancy for humans in this day and age?). HGH can be measured with a blood tests (IGF-1) or urine HGH metabolites. The good news is that if human growth hormone is low it can be given with a tiny daily needle like the needle a diabetic would use for insulin injections.

As we age we produce less melatonin, which interferes with the amount of sleep we get. It is also responsible for cortisol getting the upper hand as melatonin and cortisol are balanced among each other (read the answer under Sleep to the question: What are the nuts and bolts about sleeping?)

But melatonin can be taken at bedtime. This helps to balance your hormones and reduces your cortisol level to normal.

There are other hormones that likely are out of balance: with older age thyroid hormones are often diminished, which ages you faster. This can easily be measured, and if levels are low, it can be corrected with thyroid hormones.

Aging males often lack testosterone production, which can be determined with a blood test. If low, either bioidentical testosterone cream or a testosterone injection twice per week can be given. In women it is estrogen and progesterone deficiency that ages them prematurely. Replacement with bioidentical progesterone and estrogen cream will rebalance these hormones and slow the aging process. While the aging process affects every person, appearance can vary a great deal. Everybody is different!

In summary, I do not know the hormone status of Bill Gates. But if I were he, I would spend some money on the hormone tests mentioned. Prevention is always better than treating disease later. This is what I mean with "healing done right" (1).

Internet reference

1. Dr. Ray Schilling, 2016: "Healing Gone Wrong – Healing Done Right"
    https://www.amazon.com/gp/product/1523700904

Publications of medical questions and answers in popular magazines.

Ibtimes.com: May 20, 2017

Heart Disease and 5 Other Things That Trigger Death At Old Age

Answer by Ray Schilling, M.D., author of "Healing Gone Wrong, Healing Done Right".

Why do people die of old age?

When I was in general practice, I looked after a sizeable number of people in nursing homes. A lot of them were disabled following a stroke, heart attack or other illnesses.

I saw them on a monthly basis. Many of them died of "old age". But the real reason was not just their aging. There were underlying medical conditions that were responsible for their death.

1. Heart failure. About half of them with this condition die within 5 years despite the best medicine we used to stabilize them. This has not changed today.

2. Kidney failure. With aging there is less and less filtration capacity of the kidneys until a point in time is reached where kidney failure kills the patient. These patients' health is too fragile to consider a kidney transplant or dialysis.

3. Liver failure occurs in those patients who had too much alcohol during their life and the liver developed liver cirrhosis. Another cause for liver failure is liver cancer or liver metastases from other cancers. In obese people fatty liver disease can be followed by liver failure.

4. Brain disease: stroke is very common in old age either from hardening of the arteries or from uncontrolled high blood pressure. The older the patient is, the more devastating a stroke is. Alzheimer's disease can be another reason for premature death.

5. Bone marrow failure. With old age there is loss of some of the stem cells. This is particularly devastating in the bone marrow that has had a high turnover of cells all during the lifetime of a person. But without enough blood cells there can be bleeding from a lack of platelets, serious infections from a lack of granulocytes and lymphocytes. Some patients die of leukemia (a blood cell cancer).

6. Apart from these problems osteoporosis with brittle bones can lead to premature death. A lack of balance with old age can lead to serious falls with bone fractures. When this affects the hips, there is a high risk of mortality in the order of 50% during hip replacement surgery.

The key is to keep all your organ systems going by eating a Mediterranean diet, exercising regularly, taking vitamin D3, and replacing missing hormones (bioidentical hormone replacement therapy).

Can aging be reversed in the future?

We have been exposed to a lot of clichés about aging, which makes it more difficult to dispel rumors and to clearly focus on what can and what cannot postpone aging and the associated disabilities. Here I will attempt to summarize what is known about this topic.

The American Academy of Anti-Aging Medicine (also known as A4M) has published a book where all of this is discussed in detail (Ref.1). But there are yearly conferences as well in Las Vegas and other places where further details regarding anti-aging are discussed. Since 2009 I have been attending the conferences in Las Vegas regularly every year.

Based on this knowledge let me start by reviewing the tools of anti-aging that can be used to slow down the process of aging significantly.

1. Mitochondria

At the center of anti-aging is the preservation and metabolic optimization of the mitochondria. Each of our cells contains little particles called mitochondria, which is where our energy metabolism takes place (1). Mitochondria function like mini-batteries.

The citric acid cycle builds up ATP, which is subsequently hydrolyzed into ADP and orthophosphate releasing energy for cell metabolism (2).

Old people who shuffle when they walk and have difficulties climbing stairs have lost significant amounts of mitochondria and simply run out of energy. The key to prevent this from happening is to preserve our mitochondria. We inherited them from our mother, because only the head of the sperm, which does not contain mitochondria entered the ovum when the egg cell that was destined to become you was fertilized. Subsequently the mitochondria from mother's egg have provided all of the mitochondria in the cells of our body.

2. Preserving mitochondria

There are supplements that specifically preserve mitochondria: PQQ (=Pyrroloquinoline quinone) helps mitochondria to multiply. A typical dose to take every day is 20 mg. Mitochondrial aging is slowed down by ubiquinol (=Co-Q-10, 400 mg per day is a dose that I recommend). Co-Q-10 repairs DNA damage to your mitochondria.

There are simple lifestyle changes that you can make: eat less calories as this will stimulate SIRT1 genes, which in turn stimulate your cell metabolism including the mitochondria (3).

Resveratrol, the supplement from red grape skin can also stimulate your mitochondria metabolism. 300 to 500 mg of trans-Resveratrol once daily is a good dose.

Build regular exercise into your day – and I mean every day– as this will also stimulate your mitochondria to multiply similar to the effects of PQQ. Lipoic acid is an anti-oxidant that counters the slow-down of mitochondrial metabolism. I recommend 300 mg per day.

L-arginine is an amino acid that is a precursor of nitric oxide (NO) (4).

Red beet is a rich source of nitric oxide, which is directly released into your system. There are also commercial products for NO. This keeps the arteries open, prevents high blood pressure and also hardening of the arteries and has a direct effect on preserving mitochondria.

Researchers from the McKusick-Nathans Institute of Genetic Medicine of the Johns Hopkins University School of Medicine in Baltimore, MD found that mitochondrial DNA content varies according to age (less mitochondrial DNA in older age), sex (yes, women have more than men) and mitochondrial DNA; it even has an inverse relationship to frailty and a direct relationship to life expectancy. This paper was published in February of 2015.

Each mitochondrion has its own mitochondrial DNAcontained in 2 to 10 small circular chromosomes that regulate the 37 genes necessary for normal mitochondrial function (5).

In multi ethnic groups it was apparent that mitochondrial DNA content was dictated by the age of a person.

Frailty was defined as a person who had aging symptoms including weakness, a lack of energy compared to the past, activity levels that were much lower than before and loss of weight. When persons with frailty as defined by these criteria were identified, they were found to have 9% less mitochondrial DNA than non-frail study participants.

Another subgroup were white participants; when their bottom mitochondrial DNA content was compared to the top mitochondrial DNA content, the researchers found that frailty was 31% more common in the bottom DNA content group. This means that white people are more prone to frailty and they should take steps early on to prevent this from happening.

3. Slowing down hardening of our arteries

It makes sense that young people who do not have signs of hardening of their arteries have better blood supply to their cells and thus supply their mitochondria with more oxygen and nutrients than frail, older people. The same is true for people who exercise regularly.

Vitamin D and vitamin K2 have been shown to lower calcium in the blood vessels and to retain calcium in the bone preventing osteoporosis. This is particularly useful in postmenopausal women. This October 2014 publication mentions that apart from vitamin D and vitamin K2 resveratrol and inositol are additional factors helping to prevent heart disease and osteoporosis (6).

This September 2013 publication confirms that a deficiency for vitamin K2 is common in the general population (7).

This deficiency leads to osteoporosis and calcification of the arterial wall and causes heart attacks, strokes and bone fractures. Supplementation with vitamin K2 at 200 micrograms per day every day is recommended to prevent this from occurring.

4. Sugar and starchy foods

You need to understand that starchy foods equal sugar, once digested. As a result a refined cereal breakfast=sugar, pasta=sugar, bread=sugar, donuts=sugar, potatoes=sugar and so on. It has to do with the glycemic load (8).

When you cut out sugar and starchy foods (meaning that the glycemic index of the foods you eat is below 50) you will shed 30 to 50 pounds of weight within 3 to 5 months, if you are overweight or obese. You will feel a lot more energy. Your blood vessels will be cleaned out as the oxidized LDL cholesterol will disappear and the HDL cholesterol will mop up what cholesterol deposits were there before.

It is certainly good for you, if you are not into the sugar and candy stuff, but the seemingly harmless pizza and all the other starchy foods mentioned above are of concern as well. All of the high glycemic carbs stimulate the pancreas to produce insulin. This in turn produces inflammation in tissues including the brain. Alzheimer's disease is one of the complications of this.

Where does this leave us? For decades we have been told that saturated fats and cholesterol in our diet were the culprits, and we replaced them with sugar that is part of a low-fat diet. We need to pay attention to the glycemic index and cut out high glycemic foods. However, it is OK to eat some carbs from the medium glycemic food list and most of our carbs from the low glycemic food list. With regard to fat it is important to consume only the healthy fats like olive oil, coconut oil and omega-3 fatty acids. As you make these adjustments to your life style you will also prevent many cancers, as you normalize the body's metabolism and help prevent chronic inflammation, which can cause arthritis and cancer. Finally, pay attention to stress management. The body and the mind work together. Uncontrolled stress also leads to heart attacks and strokes.

5. Cut down on processed foods

Processed foods contain the wrong type of vegetable oils that are composed of omega-6 fatty acids. This disbalances the ratio of omega-6 fatty acid versus omega-3 fatty acids. This is typical for all the processed foods, but also fast food places in the industrialized world. The consequence of this disbalance is the formation of arachidonic acid and inflammation of tissues. This causes high blood pressure from inflammation of the arteries, arthritis from inflammation in the joints and can irritate the immune system to the point of causing autoimmune diseases. The end result after decades of exposure to a surplus of omega-6 fatty acids are disabilities from end stage arthritis, as well as heart attacks and strokes from inflammation of the arteries due to the hardening of the arteries (9).

The remedy for this is to cut out all processed food and stick to the basics of preparing your own food from healthy ingredients with no food preservatives.

Use olive oil for salads and coconut oil for cooking. Take omega-3 supplements to restore the omega-6/omega-3 fatty acid balance.

6. *Replace hormones with bioidentical ones*

When I watch postmenopausal women, many look prematurely aged with sagging skin in their faces. Had they replaced their missing hormones when they entered menopause, the bioidentical hormones used for replacement therapy would have helped their skin to remain younger looking, hardening of the arteries would have been postponed, and osteoporosis in the bones would also have been prevented (10).
With men it is now known that testosterone is vital for prevention of prostate cancer, but it is also important to prevent heart attacks, strokes and dementia as they age.
I would recommend that you see a naturopath or an anti-aging physician to have your hormones checked and, if necessary, start replacement with bioidentical hormones.

Conclusion

Slowing down aging and avoiding disabilities from aging are now a possibility, if we manage our lives in a way that the biochemistry of our bodies remains the same and our mitochondria continue to function, even when we get older. I discussed the details of how to do that above. I have also written a book on the subject of anti-aging, which deals with these topics in more detail (Book ref. 2). I hope that you incorporate at least some of these steps in your life to prevent suffering from disabilities as you age and to avoid premature aging.

Book references

Ref.1: Ronald Klatz, MD, DO and Robert Goldman, MD, PhD, DO, FAASP, Executive Editors: "Encyclopedia of Clinical Anti-Aging Medicine & Regenerative Biomedical Technologies". American Academy of Anti-Aging Medicine, Chicago, IL, USA, 2012.

Ref. 2: Dr. Ray Schilling, 2014: "A Survivor's Guide To Successful Aging":
https://www.amazon.com/Survivors-Guide-Successful-Aging-Christina/dp/1494765330/ref=sr_1_1?ie=UTF8&keywords=books+dr.+schilling&qid=1398270215&sr=8-1

Internet references

1. https://www.ncbi.nlm.nih.gov/books/NBK9896/
2. https://en.wikipedia.org/wiki/Citric_acid_cycle
3. https://en.wikipedia.org/wiki/Sirtuin_1
4. https://en.wikipedia.org/wiki/Arginine
5. https://www.ncbi.nlm.nih.gov/pubmed/25471480
6. https://www.ncbi.nlm.nih.gov/pubmed/25245999
7. https://www.ncbi.nlm.nih.gov/pubmed/24089220
8. http://lpi.oregonstate.edu/mic/food-beverages/glycemic-index-glycemic-load
9. http://www.askdrray.com/slow-down-aging-and-prevent-disabilities/
10. http://www.askdrray.com/treating-menopausal-symptoms/

    (This answer was published first here: http://www.askdrray.com/ageless-aging/).

Can aging be reversed?

While there are ways to age better with fewer diseases, we do not have scientifically proven methods to create immortality. Here I like to briefly review how to slow down aging.

1. Aging occurs because of deteriorating DNA in the center of all cells from cosmic rays and from toxins that enter the body. We also experience telomere shortening with each cell division. A telomere is the cap of each chromosome that protects the DNA. There is a limit how often a cell can divide, this is called the Hayflick limit (1).

2. The mitochondria in each cell that provide energy to the cell and thus to the body as a whole age as we get older. This aging process of mitochondria can be partially reversed with supplements like PQQ, CoQ10, L-carnitine and D-ribose.

3. As we age we lose hormone production. If we ignore this we die at the average of about 80 to 84. But if we measure hormone levels and replace what is missing with bioidentical hormones, this can add 10 to 15 years beyond the current life expectancy. With an average life expectance of 80 this makes it 90–95 of a good life without deficiencies and the feared disabilities.

4. Many people beyond the age of 60 have deficiencies in human growth hormone (HGH) production. Tests are available to establish the levels of IGF-1 through blood tests and overnight urine HGH measurements. If a person is diagnosed with HGH deficiency, this hormone needs to be replaced with a daily evening injection of HGH. This is done with a tiny needle using a pen injector, which looks similarto an insulin pen. This can add significant amounts of years, possibly between 19 and 34 years (average 26.5 years) of life according to the endocrinologist, Dr. Hertoghe from Belgium whom I heard speak at the 23rd Annual World

Congress on Anti-Aging Medicine on Dec. 13, 2015 in Las Vegas. HGH in older people has nothing to do with growth, but everything with keeping the brain and muscles active and young. It also preserves the energy for longer (2).

5. You may need some supplements to support your heart and bones: vitamin D3 (8000 IU to 10,000 IU per day), 200 micrograms of vitamin K2 per day and calcium tablets that will bring the calcium from your gut into the blood stream and further into the bone. It will also dissolve any existing calcium from the arterial walls and transport it into the bones. Not enough people know about this method of allowing your arteries to stay younger for longer and to prevent osteoporosis.

6. Never underestimate the lifestyle changes that prolong life: regular exercise, not smoking, either cutting out alcohol or reducing it to one glass of alcohol or less per day for women and two glasses of alcohol or less for men per day. This will reduce or almost eliminate cirrhosis of the liver, which significantly lowers life expectancy. Also eat a healthy diet, not the standard American diet (SAD diet). The best diet would be a Mediterranean diet with lots of virgin cold-pressed olive oil.

7. Despite all precautions, cancer remains an affliction of the aging population. Diagnose and treat cancer early! This allows curing most cancers by surgical excision. Regular colonoscopies where polyps that are found are removed right away almost completely eliminate colorectal cancer. Regular pap tests in women can eradicate cancer of the cervix. There is now a new Oncoblot test that can diagnose 25 different cancer types early.

Internet references

1. Hayflick limit - Wikipedia
2. http://www.askdrray.com/life-extended-by-several-decades/

Why is immortality impossible?

1. When we age, our hormones are not produced as much as they used to be. This ages us and does not allow our bodies to function like they did in our youth.
2. Our joints and muscles age, which leads to morning stiffness. But some people get chronic pain, stiff joints and they may need a walker or electric scooter to stay mobile.
3. Our gut does not absorb nutrients as well in old age compared to a young person. Although we can take supplements, even these may one day not get absorbed as much, as the absorption mechanism of our gut cells is failing us slowly.
4. Our brain has always been active, but in older age it is not as agile as at a younger age. We can live with some limitations. But 30% to 40% of older people develop Alzheimer's disease, and this disease ultimately kills the patient.
5. Older people have much slower filtration rates in the kidneys, which translates into less detoxification. The same is true for liver function, which slows down. As both the kidneys and the liver are our major detoxification organs, toxins can accumulate in our aging bodies. This can interfere with cell function. Intravenous chelation therapy with EDTA can detoxify the body of heavy metals like mercury, cadmium, lead etc. But this will not rejuvenate the kidney or liver tissues to do the rest of detoxification.
6. Lungs and heart are other major organs that age. When lung tissue does not absorb as much oxygen as in the past, the tissues in the body are getting oxygen deprived. The heart is very sensitive to this, but hardening coronary arteries are also an important cause of heart attacks or heart failure in older people. Without full lung function and heart function the body functions will de-compensate.

Conclusion

The more we look at wanting to achieve immortality, the clearer it gets that this is a very complex topic. I have not heard any lectures in medical school about how to achieve immortality. So, don't look at physicians and specialists to help you with achieving immortality. Regenerative medicine is a new subspecialty that at least partially attempts to help you regain some lost body function. But nobody has invented yet how to regenerate the entire body. As a result there is room for the next medical researcher population coming after us to develop this further.

Is it impossible to extend the human lifespan?

It is possible to extend human life up to about 120 to 125 years. I explained this in more detail here (1).
But it is difficult to help people to live beyond this limit, as our DNA gets so damaged in time that cell function becomes impossible. The telomeres are also shortened to the point where they will not support further cell divisions. Finally, our mitochondria, the power source within our cells, are suffering irreparable damage. And without energy we cannot live.
This is all based on our present knowledge of cell function. Future basic research into these problems may come up with newer insights. But presently these limits are there, and they keep us from reaching an age beyond 120 or 125 years.

Internet reference

1. http://www.askdrray.com/what-limits-our-life-expectancy/

Anti-aging: what are some of the best tips?

There are several factors that contribute to slowing down aging.

1. Do regular daily exercises. This elongates your telomeres, the caps of the chromosomes in each body cell. Longer telomeres have been associated with living longer.

2. Eat a Mediterranean diet. It is an anti-inflammatory diet and has been associated with longer telomeres as well.

3. Self-hypnosis, yoga, meditation and Tai Chi have been shown to produce anti-inflammatory markers in the blood and are associated with longer life and better health (1).

4. A lack of hormones at any age is bad news. When we age, we naturally tend to lose thyroid hormones (we get hypothyroidism), sex hormones (menopause and andropause), but also human growth hormone (lack of energy, development of muscle aches and pains). Here are links to what to do with testosterone deficiency (2) or what to do in menopause (3).

5. Perhaps the least understood hormone deficiency with aging is a lack of human growth hormone (4). But along with growth hormone you need to replace melatonin in the older person and watch vitamin D3 levels and the other things mentioned in the last link. Without all of these hormones and supplements you cannot delay aging as your metabolism would not be optimal, and your heart would run out of energy in the mitochondria.

Here you have it in a nutshell: these are the best anti-aging tips.

Internet references

1. http://www.askdrray.com/relaxation-reduces-inflammation/

2. http://www.askdrray.com/whats-new-about-testosterone/
3. http://www.askdrray.com/hormone-replacement-therapy-in-menopause/
4. http://www.askdrray.com/effects-of-hormones-on-the-heart/

What limits the age for a human?

Right now the limit of how old we can get is between 110 and 120 years. Occasionally you have individuals who turn a bit older. But for everybody there are limiting factors:

1. Our energy organelles, the mitochondria are disappearing as we age. Each of our body cells has hundreds of these energy packages. If only 50 % are leftover, our body energy is dwindling. The brain, the heart and the skeletal muscles have thousands of mitochondria in every cell. If half of these disappear, we fall asleep on a chair (senescent people do that) and we have a shuffled gait. Our heart may start failing, and congestive heart failure may set in.

2. Our DNA is stable most of our lives because we have repair mechanisms in place. But the older we get, the more mutations occur, as the repair mechanism ages. This can cause cancer. But we may also lose bits and pieces of our DNA, and various body deficiencies start occurring.

3. Our telomeres, the caps on each of our chromosomes, are getting shorter, the older we get. This is no problem when we are younger. But as we age, the stem cells that normally have the longest telomeres are also starting to have shorter telomeres. This affects cell replacement. If you don't replace the cells that are lacking you get organ deficiencies and organ failures. Many old people die because of heart failure, bone marrow failure (no blood cells, no immune cells), kidney failure, liver failure and dementia (brain failure).

4. Until we will be able to address these concerns expressed under point 1 to 3 we will have problems extending our life expectancy limits.

What is life like in your 70's?

I am 73 now. I feel great right now, but this is something that can wax and wane.

1. I am interested in anti-aging medicine, but I never thought that hormone deficiencies would hit me. I wrote an anti-aging book (Ref.1).

My general practitioner also has a fellowship in anti-aging medicine from the A4M.

2. He diagnosed years ago that I was thyroid deficient. It sounds easy: if there is a deficiency, hormone replacement should work. He put me on T4 thyroid hormone first, but my energy had not come back. We then tried T3 and this did not quite do it either. Finally we tried Armour (a natural T3 and T4 mix) and within two weeks my full energy had come back. But even though we had the right thyroid hormone replacement, there was a problem with the proper dosage. Once my TSH value was only 17, which meant I was hypothyroid and under dosed with regard to the replacement hormone. At that time I had back pains. When the TSH level was between 0.2 and 2.0 the back pain was gone and my energy normal. All this shows, that hormone replacement is not an open- and shut-case. It is a balancing act, and it is also important to monitor the situation. Now I go for blood tests every two months to keep an eye on the thyroid hormone levels.

3. Next I had the experience of losing my sex drive. This is not great news for a guy who enjoys his regular sex life. My testosterone level was low and my doctor said I needed testosterone replacement. We tried topical testosterone creams. But blood levels showed that the

absorption through the skin was unreliable. We switched to testosterone self-injections twice per week. This solved the problem, and my sex life was back to normal. Again, hormone replacement is not consisting of simply injecting a hormone and keeping your fingers crossed that everything is in order. Hormone levels-in this case testosterone levels- need to be monitored. I go for tests every three months.

4. My muscle aches came back a few years later, my energy was less than normal and I had problems keeping up with my daily gym exercises. So, here I thought that I was doing everything right. What happened? My doctor took an IGF-1 blood test, which indicates whether or not there is enough human growth hormone (HGH) floating around. The result was disappointing. It was low! Next I went for an overnight urine HGH metabolite test, the latest in testing for HGH deficiency. But this was also low. It meant that in my case I needed regular HGH self-injections to return to normal. After these injections were started, my muscle aches disappeared, and my endurance in the gym and my energy in general returned.

5. You sail along in life and you think that everything is going OK. I had completed two books. But then I noticed that my waterworks was not as easy as in in the past. To make a long story short: I had developed not only benign prostate hypertrophy (BPH or enlargement of the prostate), but also stage 1 prostate cancer. My PSA was elevated to 8.6. Following ablation cryotherapy of the prostate in Ft. Lauderdale by Dr. Gary Onik, an interventional radiologist, the PSA went down to around 1.0. I described all of this in detail in my third book, published in April 2017 (Ref.2).

6. Life is back to normal, but not without a new "crutch". Since my prostate surgery my sex life went downhill. But fortunately for me two little pills came to my rescue (Tadalafil and sildenafil, you may know them under the names Cialis

and Viagra). They are not covered by any prescription plan, but I don't mind paying for them myself.

7. Otherwise I enjoy the 70's. My wife and I went for extensive ballroom and Latin dance lessons since our early sixties. Now that I am retired (I retired in early 2010), we go out dancing 3 to 4 times per week, sometimes more, sometimes less. It is something I could not do easily when I was in general practice and on call at the emergency room of the local hospital. Having time and enough energy also allows us to travel-something that is not feasible when your work schedule is full.

8. I am also working on my 4th book, which will come out in early 2018 (you are reading it right now). So, life is full of twists and turns. We just have to adjust whichever way it goes. This is true for any age group, but it is necessary to never lose your oomph and your flexibility as you age!

Book references

Ref. 1: Dr. Ray Schilling, 2014: "A Survivor's Guide To Successful Aging":
https://www.amazon.com/Survivors-Guide-Successful-AgingChristina/dp/1494765330/ref=sr_1_1?ie=UTF8&qid=1398270215&sr=8-1&keywords=books+dr.+schilling

Ref. 2: Dr. Ray Schilling, 2017: "Prostate Cancer Unmasked":
https://www.amazon.com/Prostate-Cancer-Unmasked-Ray-Schilling/dp/1542880661

Chapter 3:

Alcohol

How does alcohol affect your body?

Alcohol is fat-soluble and water-soluble. It crosses the blood-brain barrier easily, which explains why people get tipsy after a few drinks. Generally speaking, alcohol is a nerve poison and a cell poison (1). Organs that are particularly sensitive to the effects of alcohol are the brain, the liver, the pancreas, the esophagus, kidneys, stomach, heart and lungs.

Common diseases associated with chronic alcohol overuse are described in this link.

But I like to briefly touch on some of these conditions. Liver cirrhosis with liver failure is a common cause of death in chronic alcoholics. Esophagus cancer can be explained directly from the toxic effect when alcoholic beverages are swallowed; the higher the alcohol percentage, the higher is the likelihood that cancer of the esophagus will develop.

The heart is very sensitive, and alcohol can have a toxic effect on the heart. This leads to "pump failure" (chronic congestive heart failure). The pancreas often gets chronically inflamed from alcohol, and this condition often leads to pancreatic cancer.

Even though cardiologists recommend 1 glass of red wine for women daily and 2 glasses of red wine daily for men to prevent heart attacks and strokes, this does not mean that alcohol has lost the toxic effects described above (2).

Internet references

1. https://www.collegedrinkingprevention.gov/specialfeatures/interactivebodytext.aspx
2. http://www.askdrray.com/what-alcohol-does-to-you/

Does beer change your body temperature?

1. Usually beer is cold when it is being served. So when you are hot and you sip on cold beer, subjectively you will feel cooler after having consumed the beer.

2. In the meantime that beer is being absorbed and metabolized. During this process your skin vessels dilate, make your skin subjectively turn warm, but you are losing heat through the skin (skin capillary dilatation and evaporation). At the same time this makes you feel hot, because when our skin is better perfused we associate this with being warm and sweaty.

3. The end result by the time the little buzz in your head has dissipated, is that objectively your body core temperature has gone down a notch. Although beer cools the body, you feel at the same time as if it would have a warming effect on your body.

Chapter 4:

Alzheimer's Disease

Could it be that sugar overconsumption causes Alzheimer's disease?

Yes, it does. Alzheimer's is called "type 3 diabetes". Here is part of a blog I wrote after listening to Dr. Pamela Smith.

At the 22nd Annual A4M Las Vegas Conference in mid December 2014 Pamela Smith gave a presentation entitled "How To Maintain Memory At Any Age". She gave a comprehensive overview of what you can do to prevent Alzheimer's disease. The better we understand the causes of Alzheimer's, the more we can interfere with the biochemical processes that lead to Alzheimer's or dementia. Various parts of the brain have different functions like pattern recognition, interpreting auditory and visual stimuli and so on (1).

In the past it was thought that once the bran is developed, it would be stationary until we die. Brain researchers have shown that instead the brain continues to develop even after the teenage years. New brain cells can develop as long as we live and new synapses, the connections between brain cells, can form all the time.

A lack of sleep causes insulin levels to rise, which causes a lack of memory. Alzheimer's disease has been termed diabetes type 3 because of this close connection of memory loss and uncontrolled blood sugar levels (2).

In fact, diabetics are three times more likely to develop Alzheimer's disease.

There are several subunits of the brain like the hypothalamus, thalamus, hippocampus and the amygdalae, which are important for normal brain function and memory (3).

The hippocampus in particular is a major memory-processing unit, which indexes, constructs and rearranges memories.

Apart from the anatomy of the brain, neurotransmitters are important for the proper functioning of the various parts. Although there are more than 100 of them the most important neurotransmitters are acetylcholine, GABA, glutamate, dopamine and serotonin. Each of these neurotransmitters binds to only one specific receptor before a signal can be sent from one neuron to the next. There is a decline in the speed of neurotransmission with age and also a memory decline. Compared to the memory in a young person a person at the age of 75 has a decline in memory function of about 40%.

Internet references

1. http://creationwiki.org/Lobes_of_the_brain
2. http://www.diabetes.co.uk/type3-diabetes.html
3. http://medicinembbs.blogspot.ca/2009/10/limbic-system.html

Why do people experience memory decline?

Apart from genetic predisposition the majority of people who come down with Alzheimer's disease do so because of neglecting the body and their brain. Neglecting elevated blood pressure by not treating it properly with medication will lead to vascular dementia (1).

As already mentioned earlier, hyperinsulinemia (too much insulin in the blood) from obesity, untreated type 2 diabetes and metabolic syndrome is another mechanism (2).

Lack of exercise is associated with a higher risk of developing Alzheimer's, and so is insomnia and a lack of sleep (less than 7 hours per night). With aging there is often poor nutrition, lack of absorption of nutrients, inflammatory bowel conditions with poor absorption of nutrients and body inflammation. A significant portion of the population is deficient for various enzymes in the methylation pathway, which can lead to high homocysteine levels and the danger of premature heart attacks and vascular dementia. Psychological health can also affect memory loss, as depression and anxiety are associated with it. Toxins like heavy metals, fuels, pesticides, solvents and fluoride can over time lead to memory loss and Alzheimer's as well.

Lifestyle habits and Alzheimer's

There are many lifestyles that cause memory loss: too much stress (from high cortisol levels that damage the hippocampus); smoking that damages acetylcholine receptors; chronic alcohol abuse leads to memory problems from the toxic effect of alcohol on brain cells, which in turn causes a disbalance of serotonin, endorphins and acetylcholine in the hippocampus.

Lack of exercise is an independent risk factor for the development of Alzheimer's disease. Exercise increases the blood supply of the brain, strengthens neural connections and leads to growth of neurons, the basic building blocks of the brain. Mood-regulating neurotransmitters are increased (serotonin, endorphins).

Sleep deprivation leads to memory loss, but so does the use of aspartame, the artificial sweetener of diet sodas (3).

Sugar consumption is the main culprit but too many highly refined carbohydrates, like white flour, pasta and white rice are equally damaging. Starches get metabolized into sugar within 30 minutes! This process causes oxidization of LDL cholesterol and plaque formation of all the blood vessels including the ones going to the brain. On the long-term this causes memory loss due to a lack of nutrients and oxygen flowing into the brain.

More details about how to preserve your memory:

Internet references

1. http://alzheimers-review.blogspot.ca/2013/11/vascular-dementia-or-alzheimers-disease.html
2. http://nethealthbook.com/hormones/metabolic-syndrome/
3. http://www.healingedge.net/store/article_neurochemical_toxins.html
4. http://www.askdrray.com/preserve-your-memory/

Which foods promote brain health?

1. The fact that the type of diet you eat has a lot to do with your brain health keeps popping up in the medical literature, and 2015 has not been any exception.

The Mediterranean diet in particular has been shown to have very positive effects on postponing Alzheimer's disease by as much as 5years (1).

2. A clinical study on 674 elderly patients (mean age 80.1 years) without dementia, was published in the journal "Neurology" (2).

It examined the question whether adherence to the Mediterranean diet would affect the degree of brain atrophy, which in turn is known to correlate with the onset of Alzheimer's disease.

The findings were interesting: a high adherence to the Mediterranean diet led to a higher total brain volume, total grey matter volume and total white matter volume as measured with high-resolution structural MRI scans. Lower meat intake led to higher brain volume and more fish intake caused the mean cortical thickness of the brain to increase. Parts of the brain that are affected in Alzheimer's patients with atrophy like the cingulate cortex, parietal lobe, temporal lobe, and hippocampus showed good volumes with the MRI scans when patients adhered to the Mediterranean diet. These volumes started to shrink when the diet was poor.

3. Those who adhered to the Mediterranean diet have brains that on MRI scan look 5 years younger and are much less likely to get affected by Alzheimer's disease. Physicians have known for a long time that people, who eat a healthy diet, exercise regularly, don't smoke and who keep mentally stimulated will generally have healthier brains than people who don't do these things.

4. What is the Mediterranean diet?

It involves eating meals that are made up of plants: vegetables, fruit, cereals, beans and nuts. You can eat fish and poultry twice per week. You cut down the amount of meat and dairy you eat, but you can have a glass of wine per day, if you like. Butter is not used for cooking, but olive oil is used instead. Here is more information of what is included in the Mediterranean diet (3).

Because there is less fat and less high glycemic index carbs in this diet, it is also a diet that lends itself for weight management (4).

You shed a few pounds and reach your ideal body mass index without paying much attention to this.

Apart from the Mediterranean diet another diet, called the MIND diet has also been shown to prevent brain atrophy (5).

This diet is a combination of the DASH diet that was developed for controlling high blood pressure and the Mediterranean diet.

5. The Mediterranean diet makes you live longer

The Nurses' Health Study that has been going on since 1976 showed that telomeres, the caps on chromosomes, were getting shorter in nurses who consumed mostly junk food (6).

Longer telomeres are associated with slower aging. And people with longer telomeres reach an older age without diseases like heart attacks, liver disease or cancer.

6. Exercise on top of the Mediterranean diet

It is not a good idea to just rely on a healthy diet, like the Mediterranean diet to prevent heart attacks, strokes and other diseases. You need regular exercise as the other ingredient to keep you well. When you combine exercise with a healthy diet your abdominal girth shrinks as this study showed (7).

Another study showed that when a Mediterranean type diet is combined with regular exercise, adult onset diabetes occurrence could be reduced by 28-59% (8).

This is quite a significant effect of two simple interventions: a healthy diet and regular exercise. Other literature has shown that Alzheimer's disease is more common in diabetics; and in those who do not have diabetes, the frequency of Alzheimer's disease is much less common.

Conclusion

Although the focus here was on diet and brain health, the most success is achieved by following a comprehensive program that involves a review of your lifestyle. This approach will be the most successful way to prevent Alzheimer's disease. It starts with quitting smoking. It goes on to starting a Mediterranean diet and staying on it. Regular exercise will take care of preventing heart attacks and strokes, but exercise also ensures that all of your brain cells continue to get oxygen and nutrients, which in turn prevents brain shrinkage. Because the Mediterranean diet has a lower calorie content than the Standard American diet, there will be weight loss until you reach your ideal body mass index. Stimulating your brain by actively working with the computer, doing puzzles, playing a music instrument, phoning friends, reading books etc. will all contribute to preventing Alzheimer's. Watching TV or movies is not an active mental activity, it is passive thinking, which means it is not as valuable as the other activities. Pick a hobby that enhances your life, and your brain will thank you for it too!

Internet references

1. http://www.cnn.com/2015/10/21/health/mediterranean-diet-healthier-brain/index.html
2. http://www.neurology.org/content/early/2015/10/21/WNL.0000000000002121
3. https://www.helpguide.org/articles/diets/the-mediterranean-diet.htm
4. https://www.cdc.gov/nccdphp/dnpa/nutrition/pdf/rtp_practitioner_10_07.pdf
5. https://www.rush.edu/news/press-releases/new-mind-diet-may-significantly-protect-against-alzheimers-disease
6. http://www.cnn.com/2014/12/03/health/mediterranean-diet-longevity/
7. https://www.ncbi.nlm.nih.gov/pubmed/26493478
8. https://www.ncbi.nlm.nih.gov/pubmed/20337844

What are the latest suggested causes of Alzheimer's disease?

1. Alzheimer's disease is caused from insulin interfering with the beta amyloid metabolism as insulin prevents the breakdown of beta amyloid. Hyperinsulinism is associated with Alzheimer's. Uncontrolled Type 2 diabetes is causing Alzheimer's (about 4-fold when compared to non-diabetic controls). Alzheimer's disease is a neurodegenerative disease of old age. We know that it is much more common in patients with type 2 diabetes where insulin levels are high (1).

Studies have shown that Alzheimer's disease can be termed "type-3 diabetes." The resulting neurofibrillary tangles and amyloid-beta deposits damage nerve cells, which are responsible for the memory loss and the profound personality changes in these patients.

2. Stress is associated with Alzheimer's: Specifically, dementia rates were 10% higher when exposed to one stressful episode, 73% higher after two stressful episodes and 151% higher when exposed to three stressful episodes (2).

3. Keep your mind busy to prevent Alzheimer's: engage in artistic activities and crafts, socialize, also stay active. If you don't use it, you lose it (3)!

4. Lifestyle: Get adequate amounts of sleep and reduce sugar consumption. Your hippocampus will thank you for it by staying alert and keeping your memory going. Don't forget to exercise regularly, particularly when you get older.

5. Replace missing hormones: an aging person has a lack of melatonin, so it is a good idea to take 3 mg of melatonin at night. If you are in andropause or menopause, see a health provider who does bioidentical hormone replacement for you. Hormones need to be in an optimal balance to allow your cell functions to be optimal.

6. How important are good genes? At the 22nd Annual A4M Las Vegas Conference in mid December 2014 Dr. Pamela Smith gave a presentation entitled "How To Maintain Memory At Any Age". She pointed out that there are about 5 genes that have been detected that are associated with Alzheimer's disease and in addition the apolipoprotein E4 (APOE4).

About 30% of people carry this gene, yet only about 10% get Alzheimer's disease, which shows how important lifestyle factors are (in medical circles this is called "epigenetic factors") to suppress the effect of the APOE4 gene (4). She also stated that our genes contribute only about 20% to the overall risk of developing Alzheimer's disease. This leaves us with 80% of Alzheimer's cases where we can use the brain nutrients and hormones discussed above and exercise to improve brain function.

7. Have adequate amounts of vitamin D3: A 2014 study showed that a low vitamin D level was associated with a high risk of dementia and Alzheimer's disease. Specifically the following observations were made (5).

Vitamin D level of less than 10 ng/ml: 122% increased risk of Alzheimer's.

Vitamin D level 10 to 20 ng/ml: 51% increased risk of Alzheimer's.

The same research group found in two trials that vitamin D deficiency leads to visual memory decline, but not to verbal memory decline (6).

Generally supplements of vitamin D3 of 5000 IU to 8000 IU are the norm now. But some patients are poor absorbers and they may require 15,000 IU per day. What the patients need in the dosage of vitamin D3 can be easily determined by doing repeat vitamin D blood levels (as 25-hydroxy vitamin D). The goal is to reach a level of 50-80 ng/ml. The optimal level with regard to nmol/L is 80 to 200 (according to Rocky Mountain Analytical, Calgary, AB, Canada).

8. I already mentioned the importance of keeping the insulin response under control under point 1. This is closely linked to cutting down your sugar consumption. An overload of refined carbs leads to an overstimulation of the pancreas pouring out insulin. Too much insulin (hyperinsulinemia) causes hormonal disbalance and leads to diabetes type 3, the more modern name for Alzheimer's. All starch is broken down by amylase into sugar, which means that anybody who consumes starchy food gets a sugar rush as well. Too much sugar in the blood oxidizes LDL cholesterol, which leads to inflammation in the body (7).

The consequences of chronic inflammation are the following conditions: hardening of the arteries, strokes, heart attacks, Alzheimer's due to brain atrophy, arthritis, Parkinson's disease and cancer.

9. The American Standard diet is the best way to get Alzheimer's disease (hamburgers, bacon and eggs, sausages, ice cream and other processed foods).

In September 2015 researchers from Rush University published results of putting Alzheimer's patients on the MIND diet. The MIND diet was a prospective study where 923 people aged 58 to 98 years participated (8).

Researchers followed these people for 4.5 years. Three groups of diets were tested: Mediterranean diet, DASH diet and MIND diet.

The MIND diet study result

The adherence to the diet was measured: those who stuck to the diet very closely, another section of participants that were less diligent, and finally one segment of people who did not take the entire thing too serious. With regard to the MIND diet the group with the highest adherence to the diet reduced the rate of Alzheimer's by 53% compared to the lowest third. This is like a highly effective Alzheimer's drug! The second group still was able to reduce the rate of Alzheimer's by 35%, which would be like a regular strength drug. The one control diets was the DASH diet (9) and the other control diet was the Mediterranean diet (10).

The group that was strictly adhering to the DASH diet reduced Alzheimer's by 39%, the group that was very conscientious in adhering to the Mediterranean diet reduced Alzheimer's by 54%. The middle thirds of both control diets did not show any difference versus the lower thirds. The conclusion was that a strict Mediterranean diet had a very good Alzheimer prevention effect, as did a strict MIND diet. However, when patients did not adhere too well to a diet, the MIND diet was superior still yielding 35% of Alzheimer's prevention after 4.5 years. The other diets, when not adhered to that well, showed no difference from being on a regular North American diet (11).

Here is more info about the MIND diet (12).

10. The newest insight is that a leaky gut can allow lipopolysaccharides (LPS) from gut bacteria to enter the circulatory system. This releases inflammatory kinins that break down the blood/brain barrier. This leads to shrinkage of the hippocampus, which is the memory center. Next the person develops dementia or Alzheimer's. Other studies have shown that obesity by itself can lead to hippocampus shrinkage (13).

Conclusion

There are several hypotheses that can explain the development of Alzheimer's. The end result is that the hippocampus is shrinking (medically call "atrophy of the hippocampus"). Too much sugar consumption leads to too much insulin production, which will interfere with the breakdown of beta amyloid. In small amounts beta amyloid is a nutrient for brain cells, in large amounts it is toxic. You can prevent Alzheimer's by eating a MIND diet or the Mediterranean diet. This was explained above. Included in this should be adequate amounts of vitamin D3 supplementation. Closely related to this is to watch your hormone status. If you are missing any hormone, replace it with bioidentical ones. Discuss this with your doctor, as you will need blood test to reach adequate vitamin D levels in your blood. Keep your mind busy, reduce stress and exercise regularly.

Note: This material was published first here (14).

Internet references

1. https://www.ncbi.nlm.nih.gov/pmc/articles/PMC2769828/
2. https://www.ncbi.nlm.nih.gov/pubmed/20488887
3. https://www.ncbi.nlm.nih.gov/pubmed/25854867
   http://www.alz.org/research/science/alzheimers_disease_causes.asp
5. https://www.ncbi.nlm.nih.gov/pubmed/25098535
6. https://www.ncbi.nlm.nih.gov/pubmed/26836174
7. http://www.news.com.au/lifestyle/food/study-links-high-sugar-diet-to-brain-shrinkage/news-story/36b2f60ffcb28cb7e102733b0a9ee195
8. https://www.ncbi.nlm.nih.gov/pubmed/25681666
9. https://www.nhlbi.nih.gov/health/health-topics/topics/dash/
10. http://www.mayoclinic.org/healthy-lifestyle/nutrition-and-healthy-eating/in-depth/mediterranean-diet/art-20047801
11. http://www.livestrong.com/article/197885-the-typical-american-diet/

12. http://www.askdrray.com/mind-diet-helps-prevent-alzheimers/
13. https://www.ncbi.nlm.nih.gov/pubmed/16216937
14. http://www.askdrray.com/what-works-against-alzheimers/

Chapter 5:

Appearance

Why do some people have chin dimples?

They are called chin dimples or cleft chin, if you want to use the more medical name (1).

We all have slight variations in regard to the development of muscles in our bodies. People with chin dimples are missing a tiny muscle in the chin area. This often runs in families. The missing muscle causes the overlying skin to retract, and you get the appearance of a dimple. There is no special deeper meaning although in the article cited above they make you believe otherwise. People with chin dimples are as normal as you or me. Let's not over-interpret slight differences in appearance!

Internet reference

1. http://www.etopical.com/chin-dimples-cause-meaning-personality-genetics-surgery-get-removal/

Chapter 6:

Arthritis

What can cause rheumatoid arthritis and how do you treat it?

Rheumatoid arthritis (RA) is an autoimmune disease where autoantibodies attack the joint surfaces. It is a multifaceted disease and typically requires that the patient needs input by a rheumatologist in order to receive optimal treatment. The standard treatment for RA is summarized in this link (1).

Before engaging in these toxic treatments, it is very worthwhile to study this link and see, if any of your food components may have triggered your arthritis (2).

Various agents in the food can contribute to the development of autoantibodies, such as wheat, soy, MSG, even salicylates. An elimination diet approach could pinpoint if there is any food component that may be the cause of your RA.

Dr. Lichten, who has treated many RA cases, has found (Ref.1, p. 85 and 86) that many patients had hormonal deficiencies, particularly a lack of DHEA when blood tests were done for this. DHEA is known to treat immune deficiencies and T-cell responses were observed to raise 10-

fold after DHEA supplementation; IGF-1 levels (an indirect measure of human growth hormone) increased and muscle mass improved when the patient exercised and used DHEA replacement. RA patients responded well to relatively low doses of DHEA (25 mg daily for women and 50 mg daily for males). Along with this Dr. Lichten sometimes found other deficiencies, like thyroid deficiencies requiring hormone supplementation. Similarly when saliva tests are done to look for sex hormone deficiencies, there may be progesterone and/or estrogen deficiency in women and testosterone deficiency in males that need to be replaced with bioidentical hormones. In RA patients there may be adrenal gland deficiency setting in, which can be diagnosed by a four-point saliva cortisol hormone test. Only these cases of true hormone deficiency will benefit from small doses of cortisol (the original bioidentical human stress hormone) given four times per day.

Here is a summary of the usual recommendations for home remedies for treating rheumatoid arthritis (3). Using electro acupuncture can be very useful for controlling chronic pain, but you still need to work out the cause for your particular case of RA (4).

Book reference

Ref. 1: Dr. Edward M. Lichten: Textbook of bio-identical hormones. ©2007 Foundation for Anti-Aging Research, Birmingham, Michigan, USA

Internet references

1. https://www.drugs.com/health-guide/rheumatoid-arthritis.html
2. https://www.rheumatoidarthritis.org/living-with-ra/
3. http://www.webmd.com/rheumatoid-arthritis/guide/default.htm
4. http://www.askdrray.com/electro-acupuncture-twice-as-effective-as-conventional-acupuncture/

What can you do about osteoarthritis?

1. For many people it is osteoarthritis that leads to chronic pain. When aging joints lose the hyaline cartilage coating, eventually bone rubs on bone. Many people think that they have to accept this condition. Conservative physicians play into that passive thinking. They wait until the pain becomes excruciating. At this point they refer the patient to an orthopedic surgeon for a total hip or knee replacement. Not so fast!

2. In the meantime, there would have been alternatives: prolotherapy, platelet-rich plasma (PRP) or stem cell therapy (1).These are newer methods that work quite well, but are often ignored by conventional physicians. If they are applied, pain often disappears and mobility returns. These patients will cancel their appointment for a total joint replacement. Besides, these surgeries often fail to give the promised relief. A conscientious surgeon will discuss the possible risks with the patient.

3. Hormone deficiencies are also often leading to muscle aches and pains. A lack of testosterone can do this to a male (andropause); a lack of estrogen and progesterone can cause muscle aches and pains to a female (menopause). Low thyroid levels will rob you of energy, make you depressed and give you aching muscles. When you looked after all of these hormones (bioidentical hormone replacement), you may still have achy muscles and joints from human growth hormone (HGH) deficiency, which can be diagnosed by a blood test (IGF-1) and a more expensive overnight urine HGH metabolite test. When this is replaced with daily injections of HGH (low dose) similar to insulin injections, the energy is likely to return, the achy muscles disappear for good and your thought processes become astute again.

4. Daily exercise is also essential to keep muscles and joints in good order, and a sensible diet like the Mediterranean diet is also important. Our bodies do best with a plant-based diet. We also need omega-3 fatty acid supplements and a good dose of vitamin D3.

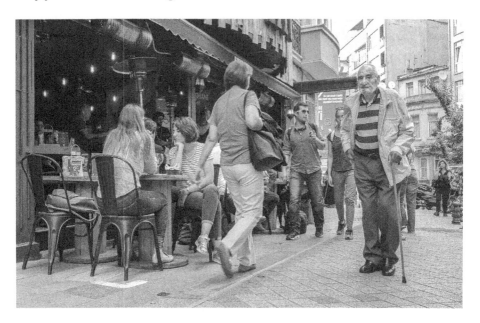

Conclusion

You don't need to have aches and pains when you get old. But if you hurt, you must think about all of your options. Think about seeing other health professionals like a naturopathic physician, an integrative medicine doctor or a regenerative medicine doctor. Medicine is moving on outside of conventional medicine. Coverall aspects if you need help. Otherwise do your part in keeping yourself healthy!

Internet reference

1. http://www.askdrray.com/prolotherapy-and-stem-cell-therapy/

How does gout develop?

Heavy consumption of beef in combination with heavy consumption of alcohol (beer, wine) leads to an acute gout attack.

Not everybody can handle uric acid in their system as well as the person next door. Some people are more vulnerable. Uric acid is one of the breakdown products of meat. We are all born with slightly different enzyme patterns. However, the person that cannot break down purines as well will end up with too much uric acid in the system until it reaches a critical point of solubility where it precipitates as uric acid crystals.

When uric acid levels exceed 7.0 mg/dL (or 0.41 mmol/L) in plasma, a critical point is reached where monosodium urate crystals, which under the microscope look like micro-needles, will be spontaneously deposited in tissue with a lack of blood supply such as tendons, joints, ligaments or cooler tissues such as ear lobes.

This point can also be reached in patients who have leukemia, lymphomas, hemolytic anemia or other cancers where purines are overproduced because of rapid cell division. Some children are born with an enzyme defect, which leads to uric acid kidney stones and severe gout and kidney damage at a young age. Most cases of gout though are in adults and are often associated with an overindulgence of meals containing large helpings of meat in combination with consumption of alcohol. This might be part of the explanation why males are much more commonly affected by gout than females (ratio of 20:1).

In the past gout was dubbed "the disease of the wealthy", as it was the affluent part of the population that could overindulge in meat and alcoholic drinks. The diet of the poor looked different: eating a roast was reserved for special occasions only. In a society of plenty, we are facing the consequences of overindulgence, and the most important point is not the pill to treat gout, but the prevention of the disease through sensible eating habits.

More info at (1).

Internet reference

1. http://nethealthbook.com/arthritis/gout/

Chapter 7:

Autism

Is it true that vaccines cause autism?

10 to 15 years ago there was a hypothesis that thimerosal, a preservative of vaccines, may cause autism. This hypothesis has been proven wrong.
1. But in the meantime due to mounting pressure from the public, most vaccines no longer contain thimerosal, the mercury preservative compound. Yet the autism rate continues to climb. This would imply that there is another mechanism that causes autism.
2. There have been large trials that showed that there is no correlation between the amount of vaccinations a child gets and autism. Vaccines Do Not Cause Autism (1).
3. This leaves the question of what causes autism? The strongest factors seem genetic factors, but there could be epigenetic factors (environmental modifications of genetic traits) that may also play a role: Research is still ongoing (2).
4. A defect in metal processing metabolism has been identified to be a cause in some with autism. Heavy Metal Metabolism in Autistic Children (3).

5. Despite all of the research there is no clear-cut answer to what causes autism and what would be an effective treatment. Many children were treated with intravenous chelation, and they improved drastically. This points to the importance of removing heavy metals from the body, because that is what chelation therapy does.

6. The next point is early intervention. Autism is treatable, but the diagnosis has to be made early, and early therapy is crucial for success. A group of DAN physicians (DAN= Diagnose Autism Now) dedicate their efforts towards diagnosis and treatment of autism.

Internet references

1. https://www.cdc.gov/vaccinesafety/concerns/autism.html
2. https://en.wikipedia.org/wiki/Causes_of_autism
3. http://www.healing-arts.org/children/metal-metabolism.htm#intro

Chapter 8:

Back Pain

Treating symptoms of back pain only is insufficient

Integrative medicine tries to treat the causes of diseases. But conventional medicine by and large still concentrates on treating symptoms.

I have written a blog about the difference of the two approaches for rheumatoid arthritis, high blood pressure, gastritis and duodenal ulcer, chronic back pain and asthma (1).

I have also written a book about "Healing Gone Wrong, Healing Done Right" (Ref.1).

In this book I am describing with many more examples how conventional medicine often makes people sick and alternative medicine methods combined with other methods can heal complicated diseases.

For instance, back pain is conventionally treated with physiotherapy and pain pills. But since the 1940's it is known that prolotherapy is quite effective in treating chronic back pain by strengthening ligaments to support the back. In the last 10 years stem cell therapy has successfully treated disc bulges and even herniated discs. Conventional medicine only offers discectomy surgery, which often makes the condition chronic. When this happens, conventional medicine offers fusion surgery. Sometimes the patient still has chronic back pain, this time from scarring. Ironically this can often be successfully treated with prolotherapy or with stem cell therapy and PRP (platelet rich plasma) to activate stem cells. This heals any joint or disc defect without scarring.

Book reference

Ref.1: Dr. Ray Schilling, 2016 "Healing Gone Wrong, Healing Done Right"
https://www.amazon.com/gp/product/1523700904

Internet reference

1. http://www.askdrray.com/treating-symptoms-not-effective-find-and-eradicate-causes/

Running on a treadmill I get lower back pain. What should I do?

A patient asked this question. The following answer would offer some advice: Don't run, rather go for a fast walk (use a treadmill setting of 4 to 4. 2 miles per hour). Secondly, see a chiropractor. You may have what they call subluxations in the facet joints that could become symptomatic with exercising. This should be assessed and treated by the chiropractor. Keep on exercising as this builds up your muscle strength, which in turn also strengthens and stabilizes your back and prevents future back injuries.

When I am angry, I tend to get lower back pain. Why is this?

Have you ever used the expression about an obnoxious person: "He or she is a pain in the back"? It is not coincidental. The lower back is an area of the body that reacts to emotions. Anxiety, anger, even depression can lead to muscle spasm in the lower back, which can be quite debilitating. I had patients like this and when a CT scan was done, the anatomy was entirely normal. Trigger point injections with a local anesthetic (like Xylocaine) will take the pain away, as it loosens up muscle spasm. A patient like this will also respond well to TENS treatments with the help of a physiotherapist. Electro-acupuncture is equally effective. A heating pad can also be helpful. Ultimately we all can benefit from more relaxation in our stressful lives. Managing stress and letting go of anger can save us a lot of grief (and backpain).

Chapter 9:

Brain

What is the dark part about the brain?

Dr. Amen, a psychiatrist and pioneer of using SPECT scans of the brain has used this technique extensively to examine various mental conditions. Dr. Amen has done many studies on people who abused drugs, marijuana or alcohol. He found that their brains show an appearance that looks like holes on SPECT scans. See the images in this link: (1). This means the brain becomes dissociated. These people cannot access adjacent brain parts that are separated through a hole. The end result is that they are impaired in their judgment, that they lose social responsibility and they injure others and/or themselves.

Dr. Amen also did many SPECT scans on drug or marijuana rehabilitated people and showed that the holes disappeared after a few months of treatment. Psychological tests could document the improvements from before and after the rehabilitation of the person.

The dark part of this is that science and mainstream medicine ignore these findings. One could use this information to motivate drug dependent people to change their behaviour pattern and agree to proper treatment. Drug dependency is extremely difficult to treat, but if people see the "hole" on the scan result, it can help in the motivation and rehabilitation process.

Internet reference

1. http://www.amenclinics.com/healthy-vs-unhealthy/alcohol-drug-abuse/

Chapter 10:

Cancer

Could the increased consumption of processed food in the past 50 years be responsible for a rise in cancer?

1. There is evidence that cancer is rising, but it may not be because of processed food. (I will get to that point below). One reason is that we are aging, and in many cases cancer is a disease of old age (1). From 50 years ago to now we have experienced an increase in life expectancy of 20 years (from age 65 to 85). A lot of faulty DNA can turn cancerous in older age where the DNA repair mechanisms get sluggish or are incomplete. This is what causes cancer, apart from habits like smoking. In smokers carcinogens are a lot more aggressive and can be responsible for various cancers. Here is a review of this subject. Why are cancer rates increasing (2)?

2. In Australia breast cancer incidence has been rising over the past decades with the mortality only slightly decreasing over the same time period. This is only one cancer type. Each cancer has its own intricacies, depending on how early it is diagnosed, how aggressive the cancer is and how well we can treat it. This determines the survival rate for a particular cancer.

3. Now to your question about processed food. The WHO has determined that a certain percentage of cancers are due to eating processed food, particularly red meat and processed meat products like sausages etc. (3) In Germany a study showed that vegetarians had 40% less cancer than meat eaters. The WHO said that dietary factors account for 30% of all cancers in the Western world and for 20% of cancers in developing countries. Those are important observations. But smoking remains the number one reason why many people get a number of cancers, not only lung cancer, but also esophageal cancer, stomach cancer, and pancreatic cancer. Red meat including processed meat accounts for some of the cases of breast cancer, colorectal cancer, prostate cancer and pancreatic cancer. But any carcinogen, either from meat processing or from smoking will contribute to the risk of developing these cancers.

You wanted to know whether the increased consumption of processed food in the past 50 years would be responsible for a rise in cancer?

• I would answer your question that part of the rise is due to the increase in life expectancy.

• But the other part is due to the fact that we consume much more processed food including red meat, sausages (beef and pork) that were labeled by the WHO to contain weak carcinogens.

• The least contribution to cancer by processed food is likely 10% (the difference between 30% of the Western world and 20% of developing countries).

• But hidden factors could bring that number up to 40% (the difference between meat eaters and vegetarians in Germany).

Internet references

1. http://scienceblog.cancerresearchuk.org/2015/02/04/why-are-cancer-rates-increasing/

2. http://scienceblog.cancerresearchuk.org/2015/02/04/why-are-cancer-rates-increasing/
3. http://www.pcrm.org/health/cancer-resources/diet-cancer/facts/meat-consumption-and-cancer-risk

Does smoking a few cigarettes cause lung cancer?

Even smoking small amounts of cigarettes can cause lung cancer and other cancers. On a population basis there is a dose-response curve, meaning the more you smoke the higher the danger of getting cancer. But individually you may for a while escape the effect of the carcinogens in cigarette smoke as antioxidant vitamins fight the effects of carcinogens to a certain extent. But don't lull yourself into thinking that you could outsmart nature!

Remember that the Framingham Heart Study was the first one to prove that cigarette smoking caused heart attacks and strokes. Other health problems are also related to it (1).

Internet reference

1. https://www.cancer.gov/about-cancer/causes-prevention/risk/tobacco/cessation-fact-sheet#q2

Is smoking cigarettes really causing cancer?

Even smoking small amounts of cigarettes can cause lung cancer and other cancers. On a population basis there is a dose-response curve, meaning the more you smoke the higher the danger of getting cancer. But individually you may for a while escape the effect of the carcinogens in cigarette smoke as antioxidant vitamins can fight the effect of carcinogens. This may be the case for a while, but the clock is ticking, and you do not mess with health.

Don't assume that you are invincible. Some people are more vulnerable than others, and you do not want to play Russian roulette with your health!

Remember that the Framingham Heart Study was the first one to prove that cigarette smoking caused heart attacks and strokes. Other health problems are also related to it (1).

Somebody may have told you that smoking cigarettes would not cause cancer because "correlation does not equal causation". You should talk to the researchers who have proven otherwise. There are literally thousands of very clever animal experiments and carcinogen toxicity studies that prove beyond a shadow of doubt that smoking cigarettes does cause cancer! So, the warning print about cancer and heart disease on cigarette packages is not something that does not apply to you and that you can blissfully ignore. It applies to everybody!

Internet reference

1. https://www.cancer.gov/about-cancer/causes-prevention/risk/tobacco/cessation-fact-sheet#q2

Is cancer caused by a lack of exercise and wrong food choices?

1. Sorry to disappoint all the exercise fans: cancer is not from a lack of exercise, although exercise will help to support your normal cell metabolism (explained below). Wrong foods may or may not have a contributory role regarding cancer development (high sugar and starch diet causing insulin response, which changes the metabolism).

2. There are many reasons for cancer and many triggers: chemicals, called carcinogens, can cause cancer.

But cancer can also be caused by oncoviruses. It can be genetically caused, which is the reason why it tends to run more often in certain cancer prone families. But Warburg has researched the metabolism of cancer almost 100 years ago, even got the Nobel price for it in 1931, and yet the elusive cancer cure has not materialized at this point (1).

3. Following Warburg's research Watson/Crick detected DNA in our cells. Ever since geneticists were fascinated by it. They also found that a cancer suppressive gene, regulated by the p53 gene could develop mutations and then cancer would occur (2). For decades this was the "in" thing. But in the last 5 to 10 years there is a revitalization of the original Warburg idea that one should concentrate on the metabolic differences between cancer cells and normal cells. This is starting to show some results.

4. Cancer cells are more acidic from lactic acid and burn glucose for energy without requiring oxygen (anaerobic pathway), while normal cells burn glucose in the aerobic pathway in the mitochondria. This difference is important. Cancer cells were found to be more vulnerable to be killed by certain manipulations.

5. Take cryoablation therapy for prostate cancer (3). The more vulnerable cancer cells are preferentially killed compared to the normal cells through a local deep freeze method. Another example is phototherapy treatment of cancer that has been used for lung cancer and esophageal cancer (4).

This method may be a lot more universally applicable than believed so far. A photosensitized dye is injected and later, when normal cells have eliminated the dye, but the defective cancer cells are still containing the dye, a laser beam kills the cancer cells preferentially, absorbing the specific laser wavelength that is specific for the dye.

6. Nobody knows which way cancer research is going. But I think it will be consumer driven: consumers want

better cures, and , and when new methods that result in better cures are emerging, these will be pushed forward, while less effective methods will become history. I think that Warburg will be revitalized and new therapies will continue to be developed from this as I indicated.

Internet references

1. https://en.wikipedia.org/wiki/Otto_Heinrich_Warburg
2. https://www.ncbi.nlm.nih.gov/books/NBK9894/
3. https://www.cancer.org/cancer/prostate-cancer/treating/cryosurgery.html
4. https://www.sciencedaily.com/releases/2015/10/151029111927.htm

Publications of medical questions and answers in popular magazines.

forbes.com: Sept. 27, 2017

How Close Are We To Curing Cancer?

Answer by Ray Schilling, M.D., author of "Healing Gone Wrong, Healing Done Right".

We are closer to a cure for cancer in 2017 than one or two decades ago, but we need to get away from using radiotherapy and chemotherapy, because the cancer stem cells are resistant to these treatment modalities.

If you want to cure cancer, you need to know about cancer stem cells (1). In my opinion, the most important breakthrough in cancer research in the last decade has been the realization that standard cancer treatment protocols don't work very well. They consisted of using surgery, radiotherapy and chemotherapy. Surgery is effective for early cancer. But radiotherapy and chemotherapy have been disappointing. Instead, cancer immunotherapy has emerged as the missing link in the last ten years. The full truth about cancer can only be understood, when we realize that most, if not all solid tumors are having their own cancer stem cells (CSC).

There are new attempts to cure cancer with low dose laser methods. Twenty patients with prostate cancer were treated with photodynamic therapy (PDT) between May and September 2014. 20% of them had a complete remission of their cancers. 35% experienced a partial remission; another 35% had no further tumor progression. In 10% the tumors progressed. These patients were given the following photosensitizers: 80 mg Chlorin E6, 10 mg Hypericin and 150 mg Curcumin intravenously. Three hours after the intravenous photosensitizers had been given, photodynamic laser therapy (PDT) was administered through a transparent catheter that allowed admission of the laser instrument up to the level of the prostate. With this approach the low-dose laser light penetrated the entire prostate gland. Three frequencies were employed that corresponded to the absorption peaks of the three photosensitizers, red light (658 nm) to activate Chlorin E6, yellow light (589 nm) to activate Hypericin and blue light (405 nm) to activate Curcumin (2).

More information here (3)

Conclusion

We are close to curing cancer in 2017. But we are not there yet. We are learning that immunotherapy will become more important to remove the last cancer stem cell. This way the cancer cannot regrow. Whether or not Dr. Weber's low dose laser therapy as described above will help is not yet determined, but it looks somewhat promising. Hopefully other non-toxic methods will be added to the cancer treatment armamentarium.

Internet references

1. http://www.askdrray.com/cancer-stem-cells/
2. http://www.webermedical.com/en/weber-medical-for-professionals/med-lasertherapy/the-new-yellow-laser/
3. http://www.askdrray.com/can-cancer-be-beaten/

Can cancer cells metabolize more glucose than normal cells?

Cancer cells have a different metabolism than regular cells. This was what Dr. Warburg investigated in the years leading up to 1931 when he won the Nobel prize for his work regarding the metabolism of cancer cells (1).

We know for a long time that there are distinct differences between the glycolytic cancer cell metabolism (Warburg effect) and the aerobic metabolism of normal cells (2).

According to the latter link it is pollution with its many chemicals that changes the cell metabolism and may cause cancer. The end result is that cancer cells ferment sugar and get energy out of this while normal cells use oxygen to go through the respiratory pathway that creates energy.

As the energy production of cancer cells through fermentation of sugar is less efficient than through the respiratory pathway in normal cells, the cancer cells use more sugar (glucose).

Internet references

1. https://en.wikipedia.org/wiki/Warburg_effect#Oncology
2. https://thetruthaboutcancer.com/otto-warburg-cancer/

Could you get cancer from makeup?

Women probably apply too many creams and lotions on their skin. Cleansers, moisturizers, foundation, powder, eye shadow, lip stick, eye shadow, eye liner, nail polish are all substances that will be in part absorbed by the user. Our skin is an organ that absorbs substances that we apply to it. If there are toxic substances- and quite a few of them are- the detoxification process takes place in the liver, and the kidneys remove the metabolic end products in the urine. As many of the chemical ingredients in these cosmetics are cancer-producing substances, it is no wonder that the liver, the kidneys and the bladder are the target organs. Read more about the dirty dozen, the chemicals in cosmetics, in this link (1).

Phthalates in the form of diethyl phthalate and dibutyl phthalate are commonly found in cosmetics and personal care products (2). They help nail polish to last longer and are industrial solvents.

In 2010 this Mexican study showed malformations in rodents after exposure of the mother to phthalates (3).

Asthmatic children were also found in another study to have absorbed higher levels of phthalates than children that had no asthma (4). As a result phthalates have been illegal in many European countries, but not yet in Canada and the US. What should you do about this? For wrinkles use a product that consists of hyaluronic acid. (I found "Pure Hyaluronic Acid Facial Serum" from Complementary Prescriptions, Carson City, NV, and Yu InfiniSerum, a cream manufactured by Nutrazyne Research LLC, Highland, UT). Between both of those non-toxic skin applications you likely will not need any other cosmetics on your skin. If you feel you do, insist on natural ingredients that do not irritate your skin. Do you really need a lipstick? If you do, make sure to avoid products that contain lead or other cancer producing metals as this was discussed recently on the news (5).

More info about the subject in this link (6).

Lip sticks also have dangerous chemicals in them like parabens and lead as reviewed here (7).

Internet references

1. http://www.davidsuzuki.org/issues/health/science/toxics/dirty-dozen-cosmetic-chemicals/
2. https://www.thoughtco.com/are-phthalates-in-cosmetics-dangerous-1204027
3. https://www.ncbi.nlm.nih.gov/pubmed/20368132
4. https://en.wikipedia.org/wiki/Phthalate#Health_effects
5. http://www.cbsnews.com/news/toxic-metals-and-cancer-risks-found-in-lipsticks-lip-glosses/
6. http://www.askdrray.com/toxins-in-the-bathroom/
7. http://www.askdrray.com/lead-still-poisoning-us/

Can cancer ever be turned into a disease we can live with?

We are talking about cancer, as if it would be one disease. The only common factor with respect to cancer is that at the end stage there is uncontrolled cell division, which leads to premature death.

In reality there are important differences between cancers, which often is parent when a particular treatment modality works for one type of cancer, but the same method will not work for others. Oncologists keep track of these differences and try to figure out the best treatment modality for each cancer type and also for the stage of cancer, which is found on initial examination.

1. Prostate cancer has experienced an increase in survival since the introduction of PSA screening and improvements in the treatment methods. While the standard radical prostatectomy has 10-years survival rates of about 75%, there are newer methods with a 10-year survival rate of 100% and recurrence rate of only 6%. I explained this in this link (1).

2. A modified smallpox vaccine has been used in advanced cancer patients and significant improvements were observed despite the late stage of their cancer (2).

3. Testicular cancer and germ cell tumors belong into the hands of an experienced urologist with input from a major Cancer Center. 5-year survival statistics for testicular cancer for stage 1, 2 and 3 are now at 98%, 93% and 61%. Germ cell tumors have a cure rate in 5 years of 76%, 50% and 42% for stages 1, 2 and 3. It might help to be reminded that in the 1970's the 5-year survival for mediastinal germ cell tumors was only 3% for all stages! These improvements have been possible because of the use of chemotherapy for the later stages and the orchestration following the initial orchiectomy with post surgical radiotherapy of the paraaortic lymph nodes for the earlier stages (3).

Conclusion

It is an uphill battle to improve survival rates for various cancers. Each cancer type has its own hurdles to be overcome, and one treatment modality is not suitable for all. But as these examples show, real progress is possible. We need to use cancer prevention methods much more vigorously, if we want to turn cancer into a type of disease that we can control and "can live with".

Internet references

1. http://www.askdrray.com/prostate-cancer-treatment-is-often-inadequate/
2. http://www.ctvnews.ca/canadian-made-virus-shows-promise-as-cancer-treatment-1.690978
3. http://nethealthbook.com/cancer-overview/testicular-cancer/treatment-testicular-cancer/

I have a lump in the esophagus; I find it progressively more difficult to swallow. Must I seek the advice of a physician, when I know that esophagus cancer cannot be treated?

1. Don't play physician with yourself. When I am sick, I have to seek the advice of a physician even though I would be medically qualified. But you will be biased when you try to diagnose yourself. This goes for anybody.

2. I suggest you get a referral to a gastroenterologist. You will need an esophagoscopy to see what is going on in your esophagus. Persons can develop esophageal diverticula that can feel like a lump, but are different. It is premature to come to a diagnostic conclusion. You need to see the gastroenterologist first.

Is there a method that will only kill cancer cells, but not normal cells?

That's a question oncologists have been thinking about for decades. Chemotherapy and radiotherapy do not fit into that category of destroying only cancerous cells, but not normal cells. Lately there has been an interesting observation, which I described in my 2017 book (Ref.1).

Prostate cancer develops from prostate cancer stem cells. The same principle is true for many other solid tumors. The reason radiotherapy and chemotherapy are not successful on the long term is that these cancer stem cells are very resistant to chemotherapy and radiotherapy. Then, when no more therapy is given, these cancer stem cells start multiplying and oncologists call this a resistant tumor.

There are two methods that I am aware of that may kill cancer stem cells, but not normal cells.

1. Ablation cryotherapy for prostate cancer: This is a method where tumor cells are frozen with a special Argon sound, which is verified with temperature gages. Repeated freezing and thawing is necessary to ensure that all the cancer cells and prostate cancer stem cells are killed. Another technique called IRE surgery or NanoKnife (irreversible electroporation), which was developed by Dr. Onik. It can be combined with the cryosurgery. Both of these methods will kill prostate cancer stem cells and this is the reason there are no recurrences. There is an additional effect: both of these methods stimulate the immune system to produce killer T cells that wipe out any remaining cancer cells. When the prostate cancer stem cells are dead, any former inhibition of the immune system (from the cancer stem cells) is nullified. This is a tremendous help especially in more advanced prostate cancer.

2. Photodynamic therapy of a group of inoperable prostate cancer patients: 20 patients with prostate cancer were treated with photodynamic therapy by Dr. Weber in Germany. The treatments took place between May and September 2014. 20% of them had a complete remission of their cancers. 35% experienced a partial remission; another 35% had no further tumor progression. In 10% the tumors progressed. These patients were given the following

photosensitizers: 80 mg Chlorin E6, 10 mg Hypericin and 150 mg Curcumin intravenously. Three hours after the intravenous photosensitizers had been given photodynamic laser therapy (PDT) was administered through a transparent, permanent catheter that allowed admission of the laser instrument up to the level of the prostate. With this approach the low-dose laser light penetrated the entire prostate gland. Three frequencies were employed that corresponded to the absorption peaks of the three photosensitizers, red light (658 nm) to activate Chlorin E6, yellow light (589 nm) to activate Hypericin and blue light (405 nm) to activate Curcumin (1). In addition to PDT patients also received an immunostimulator preparation, called Gc protein-derived macrophage activating factor (GcMAF). This is described under this link (2).

Finally, in order to take advantage of the minimal differences regarding poor oxygenation of cancer cells versus good oxygenation of normal tissues, intravenous oxygen was given with the oxygenation system of the German company Oxyven (3).

This strengthened the normal tissue and weakened the cancer tissue.

Conclusion

There are newer methods as described above that may solve the old question whether it is possible to destroy only cancerous cells, but not normal cells. Dr. Onik in Ft. Lauderdale has made very solid progress with the combined NanoKnife surgery and ablation cryotherapy for prostate cancer. Dr. Onik has done 10-year survival data with 100% survival and only 6% recurrences.

Dr. Weber in Germany has pushed low-dose multi-colored laser therapy to the point where some incurable cancer patients have been cured. In comparison to Dr.

Onik's data Dr. Weber's laser therapy requires a long-term trial with 10-year survival data.

More info: Can cancer be beaten (4)?

Book reference

Ref. 1: Dr. Ray Schilling, 2017: "Prostate Cancer Unmasked" https://www.amazon.com/Prostate-Cancer-Unmasked-Ray-Schilling/dp/1542880661

Internet references

1. http://www.webermedical.com/en/weber-medical-for-professionals/med-lasertherapy/the-new-yellow-laser/
2. https://www.ncbi.nlm.nih.gov/pubmed/14666733
3. https://www.youtube.com/watch?v=qWRhxw9cH7U
4. http://www.askdrray.com/can-cancer-be-beaten/

If old age or disease won't kill you, will cancer do it?

Yes, the common diseases that kill a person in old age are heart attacks, strokes, Alzheimer's disease and cancer. Cancer is a disease of the aging person. It is so, because DNA mutations happen more often as we age. On the other hand, if we diagnose cancer in stage 1 or 2 (in the early stages), it is quite often curable.

One of the new criteria that is lesser known is the fact that there is a very sensitive cancer blood tests, called the Oncoblot test (approved about 3 years ago by the FDA).

If physicians use this blood test for the early diagnosis of cancer and treat the cancer right away, the patient has a good chance to live several years longer. As we age, we may come down with another cancer down the road, but it cannot be emphasized enough that it is early diagnosis and treatment that helps the patient live longer. Churchill coined the phrase to "Never, never give up ..." It applies to persistent prevention and diligent treatment as well.

1. Coffee cannot cure cancer, but a large study found the following (1):
• Less than 1 cup of coffee per day: 6% lower death rates than non-coffee drinkers.
• 1 cup to 3 cups of coffee per day: 8% lower death rates.
• 3 to 5 cups of coffee per day: 15% lower death rates.
• More than 5 cups of coffee per day: 12% lower death rates. Incidentally, it is the antioxidants in the coffee that are beneficial. But green tea does have very similar health benefits!

2. Next, what does cinnamon do? Cinnamon is a gentle immune stimulator (2).

This may be enough to help you together with healthy food habits and exercise to prevent cancer, but it will not be enough by itself to CURE cancer. Curing cancer is a completely different matter. Even coffee consumption together with cinnamon won't cure a single cancer! There are a lot of sensationalist "medical websites" which promise incredible cancer cures, citing everything from curcumin to mangosteen or apple cider vinegar; but be aware of false information! There is no "magic bullet"!

Internet references

1. http://www.askdrray.com/coffee-could-be-a-lifesaver/
2. https://www.thesuperfoods.net/cinnamon/cinnamon-for-the-immune-system

Why are cancer cells so difficult to identify; are there no cell markers that would give them away in at test?

1. For the past 3 years the Oncoblot test has been available (1). This blood test can analyze 25 of the common cancer cell types in one test.
2. I had my prostate cancer tested this way before the PSA level went higher. As a result I could get ablation cryotherapy done earlier when it is more likely to be curative. 2 months after the prostate surgery the Oncoblot test was repeated and was negative. My PSA test also went down from 8.6 ng/ml to around 1 ng/ml, which according to my interventional radiologist means the cancer is gone.
3. The Oncoblot test is a test that checks for a genetic marker, the ENOX2 proteins from cancer cells, exactly what you had thought about. With this test the difference between normal cells and cancer cells is being exploited for cancer screening.

Internet reference

1. http://www.askdrray.com/catch-cancer-early/

Why can cancer still not be cured? When will this change?

We are able to cure quite a few cancers, provided they are detected early enough. Here are a couple of points worth noting about this.
1. With early detection all of the cancer can be removed and it won't return down the road. In this context it is important to recognize that every cancer has its own cancer stem cells. If they are removed with the tumor, there

will not be any cancer recurrence in the future. If cancer stem cells are left behind, there will be a recurrence of the cancer (1).

2. When cancer is more advanced than stage 1 or 2, it is difficult to cure cancer with only surgery. There are local metastases or distant metastases present that will often not respond to chemotherapy or radiotherapy.

3. Some of the cancers that have been successfully treated are skin cancer, cancer of the cervix, colon cancer (when colonoscopies were done regularly and you detect early colon cancer), breast cancer (early stage), prostate cancer (stage 1 and 2). The problem is though, as pointed out under point 1, that the cancer must be detected early.

4. One important tool for the physician that came out about 3 years ago is the Oncoblot test, capable of diagnosing 25 different cancers early (2). I have explained this in more detail under this link. In my own case of prostate cancer it was the Oncoblot test that prompted me into action, and fortunately for me ablation cryotherapy was able to get rid of my cancer and I am prostate cancer free. The Oncoblot test picks up developing cancers 7 to 8 years before other diagnostic methods can detect it. This combined with early surgical removal of any cancer is likely the future of cancer medicine. It is all about early detection and early treatment!

Internet references

1. https://en.wikipedia.org/wiki/Cancer_stem_cell
2. http://www.askdrray.com/catch-cancer-early/

Cancer is difficult to treat, is it a supernatural disease?

It seems that cancer is a difficult disease to treat. But there are a few facts we need to become aware of before we make that statement.

1. Not every cancer is caused by the oncoviruses, carcinogens or a gene abnormality. There is a lot of diversity among various cancers.

2. It is not too long ago that cancer stem cells have been detected. The news about cancer stem cells is that they are very resistant to chemotherapy and radiotherapy (1). But what are oncologists doing when they treat more advanced cancer? They use radiotherapy and/or chemotherapy, which does not make sense.

3. Immunotherapy for cancer is emerging as a new subspecialty (2). But we do not know all of the answers yet for all of the cancers.

4. The key in any cancer treatment is to detect cancer early. As mentioned before, the Oncoblot test is a new tool that can be used to diagnose cancer early. This is described here (3). It can pinpoint, where a cancer is starting. Further tests, such as MRI studies can show more.

5. Next, early cancer excision is the treatment of choice for most stage 1 and stage 2 cancers (there are 4 stages of cancer). I described prostate cancer treatment before: ablation cryotherapy and the use of the nano knife (4).

6. Close follow-up investigations are important to make sure the cancer does not come back. A repeated Oncoblot can provide the answer, and there are other blood tests as well. Sometimes a repeat surgery has to be performed, if there is a recurrence. In future some of the immunological procedures might be contemplated.

Conclusion

I don't think that cancer is a "supernatural disease". It is more difficult to handle than some of the other illnesses that affect us. When it comes to cancer it is important to diagnose it early, treat it while it is in stage 1 or 2 (also early) and to monitor progress after the treatment. Ablation cryotherapy in combination with IRE/NanoKnife surgery is also a strong stimulus of the immune system, which can wipe out any remaining cancer cells left behind. It is a form of immunotherapy.

More info on cancer stem cells here (5).

Internet references

1. https://www.ncbi.nlm.nih.gov/pmc/articles/PMC4021765/
2. http://blog.dana-farber.org/insight/2015/05/the-science-of-pd-1-and-immunotherapy/
3. http://www.askdrray.com/catch-cancer-early/
4. http://www.askdrray.com/prostate-cancer-treatment-is-often-inadequate/
5. http://www.askdrray.com/cancer-stem-cells/

Is there a "sour honey cure" of cancer?

1. Something as major and complicated as these Simple home remedies like sour honey, lemon vinegar juice, alkaline diets and other such claims cannot cure a complex disease like cancer. A lot of unscrupulous individuals peddle "miracle cures", taking advantage of the plight of the cancer patient and their families and bilking them of their money.

2. Cancer itself is complicated with radio-resistant and chemotherapy resistant stem cells and mature cancer cells. Conventional cancer therapy may destroy the regular cancer cells, but leave the cancer stem cells behind from which new cancer cells develop.

3. Surgery in the early cancer stages is successful curing cancer as it removes both mature cancer cells and cancer stem cells. Ablation cryotherapy also works for early cancer. Another method, called the NanoKnife also destroys both cancer cells and cancer stem cells (1).

4. Cancer is a complicated topic, there are no simple remedies, and prevention is crucial: stop smoking, cut out sugar and starch, take vitamin D3 and fish oil supplements and exercise regularly.

Internet reference

1. http://www.askdrray.com/prostate-cancer-treatment-is-often-inadequate/

Publications of medical questions and answers in popular magazines.

apple.news: May 12, 2017

Why Is Cancer So Common and How Can We Reduce Our Risk?

Answer by Ray Schilling, M.D., author of "Healing Gone Wrong, Healing Done Right".

We have a higher life expectancy than a few decades ago. As cancer is a disease of older age, we are at a higher risk of getting cancer, the older we turn.

On the other hand, there is a lot more known about cancer now than in the past and we can lower our risk by utilizing this knowledge.

• Cancer is one of the conditions where there is a strong association to chronic inflammation in the body. Chronic exposure to smoking causes a transition into chronic bronchitis and eventually emphysema. As cigarette smoke also contains carcinogen (cancer producing chemicals), a close link has been established between cigarette smoking and lung cancer. Similar transitions have been observed with cancer of the cervix and exposure to human papillomavirus infections that by themselves can be asymptomatic. Eventually the chronic inflammation of the tissue around the cervix leads to cancer of the cervix. Cancer of the pancreas is another example. Here there is a transition from chronic pancreatitis (often started by exposure to chronic alcohol abuse) to cancer of the pancreas. Finally there is the example of the transition from liver cirrhosis to liver cancer. The more severe cirrhosis of the liver is and the more chronic inflammation there is in the liver, the higher the risk to develop liver cancer

• Here are some anti-inflammatory steps you can take: Start eating the Mediterranean diet, which is an anti-inflammatory diet; the Standard North American diet is carcinogenic (cancer producing). Eat more vegetables, avoid sugar, avoid processed foods and you are already a lot healthier and cancer resilient! Add to that antioxidants like resveratrol, vitamin C, molecularly distilled fish oil (two capsules twice per day) and 5000 IU of vitamin D3 daily. These are anti-inflammatory supplements that keep you out of trouble.

• Regular exercise leads to better tissue perfusion and stimulation of the immune system. Oxygen penetrates all of the tissues right down to the cellular level. This prevents glycolysis in cells that do not get enough oxygen from prolonged sitting and inactivity. Mortality is getting significantly reduced when cancer patients exercise (1).

• Green tea extract is an established natural substance and beneficial antioxidant. But now it has been found that green tea extract kills oral cancer cells. It does not have the usual side effects that chemotherapeutic agents have. Yet it seems effective in killing oral cancer cells. Fortunately for the patient, the normal cells stay unharmed. As a

result there are no stomach upsets, there is no loss of hair and no immune suppression. Green tea extract may also be effective against other cancers (2). Further ongoing research will investigate this.
- Cancer rates go up after menopause and andropause. In men andropause, the equivalent of menopause is easy to spot and treat. It is about a lack of testosterone, which is confirmed with a blood test and treated with testosterone until the blood level comes back to normal and the symptoms disappear (lack of drive, loss of erections). In women symptoms of menopause are more subtle, but more profound when they have fully developed. Symptoms of hot flashes, night sweats and vaginal dryness have all been found to be strong predictors of menopause. FSH and LH hormones are above the normal range when a woman is in menopause and this is a very reliable test for menopause that your doctor can order. Usually in menopause it is the progesterone that is no longer produced by the body because the woman stopped ovulating and her ovaries do no longer produce progesterone in the missing corpus luteum that would have followed ovulation. Treatment of menopause involves mostly replacing missing progesterone with either the oral FDA approved versions, as Prometrium (100 mg capsules) taken at bedtime or as bioidentical progesterone cream (from compounding pharmacies), which is applied to the skin. Some women do require an additional small amount of estrogen (as BiEst cream applied to the skin) to rebalance her hormones. Not every physician is comfortable with bioidentical hormone replacement. Most naturopaths are familiar with this. The reason this is important is that your body function returns to normal and your cancer risk is going down compared to those who don't replace hormones. More info available in my book: "Healing Gone Wrong – Healing Done Right". (3).

- Stress plays an important role not only in cardiovascular disease (heart attacks and strokes), but also in the development of cancer. An overproduction of cortisol leads to a relative lack of melatonin, which is important to maintain a healthy immune system. You can rebalance your hormones by relaxation methods like yoga, self-hypnosis and meditation (4).

Conclusion

As I mentioned above, there are a number of factors that in combination can lead to cancer. We cannot do anything about aging, which is an independent risk factor for developing cancer. But we can reduce inflammation, stimulate our immune system and keep in shape with exercise. We can keep our hormones balanced even beyond andropause and menopause by using bioidentical hormone replacement. Relaxation methods can help us to keep our immune system strong. Whatever you do, start with an anti-inflammatory diet like the Mediterranean diet. Add to this regular exercise and take the supplements indicated. This way you can minimize the risk of getting cancer.

Internet references

1. http://nethealthbook.com/news/exercise-curbs-cancer/
2. http://nethealthbook.com/news/green-tea-extract-kills-oral-cancer-cells/
3. https://www.amazon.com/gp/product/1523700904
4. http://nethealthbook.com/health-nutrition-and-fitness/fitness/stress-management-relaxation-techniques/

Is it true that oncologists, if they come down with cancer themselves, will refuse chemotherapy?

The newest information about chemotherapy is that cancer stem cells are resistant to it. The second important new information is that cancer stem cells are also radiotherapy resistant. This means an advanced cancer that is treated with chemotherapy and radiotherapy can regrow the moment the treatment is finished.

If you want to cure cancer, you need to know about cancer stem cells. In my opinion the most important breakthrough in cancer research in the last decade has been the realization that standard cancer treatment protocols don't work very well. They traditionally consisted of using surgery, radiotherapy and chemotherapy. Surgery is effective for early cancer. But radiotherapy and chemotherapy have been disappointing. Instead cancer immunotherapy has emerged as the missing link in the last 10 years. The full truth about cancer can only be understood, when we realize that most, if not all solid tumors, are having their own cancer stem cells (CSC). In the past this was only recognized for leukemia, largely because of a lack of testing methods for solid tumors. We now have at least two methods of proving the existence of CSCs in solid tumors, as I will explain in more detail below. Using this new cancer stem cell concept, cancer can only be cured when the CSCs are eradicated.

New assays for cancer stem cells

1. Originally the concept of regular stem cells was proven in mice by radiating them and injecting bone marrow cells into them to rescue them (1). When the animals were sacrificed colonies were detected in their spleens that were of the same cell type as the injected stem cells. This new thinking revolutionized the treatment of leukemia. Bone marrow transplants were introduced that allowed in some

cases a cure for leukemia. Presently there is a new wave of stem cell treatment applications for a variety of conditions, mostly non-cancer applications.

2. With regard to developing an assay for cancer stem cells in solid tumors researchers took a strain of hairless mice that are known to be immune deficient (they lack thymus derived lymphocytes or T cells). They are officially called "nude mice" (2).

When human cancer stem cell samples are injected into them, they develop the original cancer of human origin, and they succumb to metastases. Histologically the tumors in these mice are the same as the original human cancer.

3. Another mouse model was also shown to be equally effective in demonstrating CSC activity. The immune system of regular laboratory mice can be paralyzed with prior chemotherapy treatment. Using these chemotherapy pre-treated mice the CSC assay works very similar to the one using nude mice (3).

If isolated cancer stem cells are injected into the nude mouse or immunosuppressed mouse model, cancer cells, such as prostate cancer cells will grow in a short time that look histologically the same as prostate cancer found in prostate biopsies from a man affected by prostate cancer.

Conclusion

I do not know whether or not it is true that 9 out of 10 oncologists would not use chemotherapy, if they had cancer themselves. But when you think about the fact that cancer stem cells won't respond to chemotherapy, this makes actually sense. It is a well known fact that chemotherapy has disastrous side effects for the patient. It would be better for these oncologist to use an immunostimulation therapy, the NanoKnife or irreversible electroporation (IRE) or the ablation cryotherapy as pointed out here (4).

More info about cancer stem cells (5).

Internet references

1. http://stemcellfoundation.ca/en/about-stem-cells/canadas-contribution/
2. https://en.wikipedia.org/wiki/Nude_mouse
3. https://www.ncbi.nlm.nih.gov/pmc/articles/PMC2827660/
4. https://www.roswellpark.org/article/nanoknife-offers-aggressive-promising-treatment-option-locally-unresectable-pancreas
5. http://www.askdrray.com/cancer-stem-cells/

Warning signs for cancer

With early prostate cancer there are very few indications that you are having this cancer.

1. I had a low PSA (=prostate specific antigen) blood level at around 3.0, which may have been due to a prostate enlargement (prostate hypertrophy). At the anti-aging conference in Dec. 2015 in Las Vegas I heard about a new sensitive blood test that monitors for 25 different cancer types including prostate cancer (1).

2. I had this test done and it was positive for prostate cancer. I scheduled for a 3-dimensional prostate biopsy with the interventional radiologist, Dr. Gary Onik from Ft. Lauderdale, FLA. This confirmed a stage 1c prostate cancer. We repeated the PSA test and ironically it was now clearly elevated at 8.6.

3. I had ablation cryotherapy and NanoKnife surgery, which removed all of the prostate cancer (2). Following the surgery the PSA level went down to 1.0 and the Oncoblot

repeat test was negative for prostate cancer. The reason I went to Dr. Gary Onik is that he had done a 10-year follow-up on a group of about 70 prostate cancer patients. 100% survived. 6% of them had a cancer recurrence. This was the best survival statistics I could find in the literature.

    4. I wrote a book about what I found with my literature review. It also contains the exact procedure that was done on me (Ref.1).

    5. My repeat PSA tests have been unchanged since my surgery in August 2016.

    6. This is just one example for the development of prostate cancer. However there are early warning signs for other cancers. For the prevention of breast cancer regular self-examinations are crucial. Even a tiny lump should never be ignored! Mammography can be used to detect early lesions, and an ultrasound of the breast is a valuable test. If a lesion is found, biopsies can determine, whether the lesion is benign, and surgical intervention is possible at an early stage.

Book reference

Ref. 1: Dr. Ray Schilling, 2017: "Prostate Cancer Unmasked": https://www.amazon.com/Prostate-Cancer-Unmasked-Ray-Schilling/dp/1542880661

Internet references

1. http://www.askdrray.com/catch-cancer-early/
2. http://www.askdrray.com/prostate-cancer-treatment-is-often-inadequate/

Chapter 11:

Contraception

Can she get pregnant, if he pulled it out, cleaned it and reinserted it again?

Yes, it is possible that she gets pregnant. The reason is that sperm are hiding inside the urethra. So, you think "all clear" because you wiped it off. And nature says "tricked you", because you massage it all over her cervical opening when you come back in and it dribbles sperm. The mucous of the cervix has a remarkable ability to attract sperm and make them swim against the stream up into the Fallopian tubes where an egg is waiting to be fertilized. For anybody who has not heard it yet: "the pull and pray" approach does not work!

Can I get pregnant, if he just inserts his penis?

At least have him use a condom before he inserts his penis. This gives you a security factor of 75% to 85% to avoid pregnancy. A male can leak sperm, even before he ejaculates, and even in the "pre-cum" viable sperm cells can be found.

Contraception methods exist. Read up on the various methods and decide and what would be right for you. If you are young, but want to have kids later in life, the birth control pill would probably be best for you. Discuss this and the pros and cons with your physician.

How does a married couple avoid pregnancy when they have sex?

Couples who have regular sex have the same problem as single people who have sex. If you have unprotected sex, you can get pregnant.

Couples use barrier methods (condoms, female condoms) and the birth control pill for awhile. But when they want to get kids, they use nothing. They start discussing what permanent contraceptive method they want to use on the long term. They also have to decide, how many children they can raise. Economical considerations play as much of a role as health considerations. Studies have shown that children from larger families feel more comfortable with more kids than others.

The decision what to do when you want something permanently done is strictly between the couple. Some couples prefer that the man has a vasectomy. Another couple decides that she wants a tubal ligation. If the husband had a vasectomy, it is important to still use condoms until he gets the "all clear" signal from the doctor in the form of a negative sperm test at three months after the procedure. Vasectomy and tubal ligation have the advantage that once the procedure is done the couple no longer has to think about contraception. You can just concentrate on enjoying sex. Beside that sex is healthy (1).

Internet reference

1. https://www.healthline.com/health/healthy-sex-health-benefits#overview1

Chapter 12:

Death

Why do people die of old age?

1. People die of cardiovascular disease (strokes and heart attacks), of cancer and of essential organ failure (liver, kidneys, lungs, brain, heart, bone marrow).

2. On a cellular level it is because our DNA is aging and has mutations that render the genes ineffective. When genes cannot fully express themselves, there is loss of body function. The mitochondria are also aging. They drop off in number, but they are also not functioning as well as in younger age. Mitochondria are the powerhouses of our cells. We cannot live without them. Here are some causes of Death in Adults with Mitochondrial Disease.

All the essential organs have lots of mitochondria in their cells, so these organs that we rely on as essential organs will start failing in their function. This is how heart failure, lung failure, kidney failure, Alzheimer's diseases (brain failure), liver and bone marrow failure develop.

3. It depends now on the explanation you like best for the reasons why people die of old age. Clinically it is because of the various organ failures. It is the weakest organ that stops functioning properly because of DNA

aging, telomere shortening and because of losses of mitochondria and malfunctioning mitochondria. At the bedside of a dying patient you will not see the microscopic aspects. You see weakness, frailness and finally death taking over. Sometimes it is difficult to explain things the way they are. From a clinical point of view there is a patient with a failing organ, which later leads to death. But at the same time underlying all of this are these complex aging phenomena of DNA mutations, mitochondrial malfunction and telomere shortening.

This is all happening at the same time when people die of old age.

Internet references

1. https://www.ncbi.nlm.nih.gov/pubmed/26354038
2. http://learn.genetics.utah.edu/content/basics/telomeres/

Chapter 13:

Depression

Will my depression ever go away? I have tried drugs and exercise, but nothing seems to work. Sometimes I am suicidal.

First I like to answer the question you asked initially:

1. Depression can be complicated. If you take antidepressant medicine, this may help for a low serotonin or low dopamine level in the brain. But it will not help against the "stinking thinking" that is going on in your mind. You need cognitive behavioural therapy for that.
2. Exercise and socializing are marginally effective against depression, but this is obviously not enough for your depression.

Let's talk about depression in general

Depression is common: 10% of all men and 20% of all women have a period of depression in their lives. In people with medical illnesses depression is more common: 20% to 40% (Ref.1).

The peak age for depression is usually the age of 25 to 44. There are special groups where depression is also common. In adolescents 5% are affected with depression and 13% of women tend to get depressed after delivery, a condition called postpartum depression.

In any age group there is a risk of suicide when people are depressed, but with adolescents this is particularly true.

About 10% to 15% of people with general medical illness are developing depression, such as patients with Parkinson's disease, stroke, Alzheimer's disease, cardiac disease, HIV infection, end-stage renal failure and cancer.

Causes of depression

Officially, it is not known what causes depression. That is what medical textbooks say. However, other books like Datis Kharrazian's book "Why isn't my brain working?" offers several scenarios that can cause depression and he has examples of cases that were cured of depression (Ref.2). He points out that deficiencies in two major brain transmitters can cause depression: serotonin and dopamine.

1. Serotonin is produced in the midbrain from the amino acid tryptophan in two biochemical steps. These biochemical conversions require iron, vitamin B6, vitamin B12, niacin, folic acid and magnesium as co-factors. But you also need the "large neutral amino acid transporter" (LNAA) to transport tryptophan through the blood/brain barrier into the brain.

2. Dopamine is a neurotransmitter that is produced in the frontal lobes of the brain. It is also necessary for learning. Dopamine is synthetized by the brain from tyrosine, which has to be manufactured in the liver from the amino acid phenylalanine. You need to have a healthy liver to produce tyrosine, which needs to be transported through the blood/brain barrier into the brain; similar to

tryptophan this requires the "large neutral amino acid transporter" (LNAA). People with hepatitis, fatty liver, insulin resistance or diabetes may have problems with the LNAA transporter, which can cause dopamine deficiency (Ref.2). But as mentioned earlier they may also have low serotonin because tryptophan was not transported into the brain. This will happen with sugar overconsumption, as insulin resistance develops and affects the LNAA transporter resulting in both low serotonin and dopamine (Ref.2).

3. Since the 1990's it is known that inflammation is also a possible factor in the causation of neurological disease including depression. Ref. 2 points out that gut issues can become brain issues as inflammatory substances can leak through a leaky gut into the blood stream and trough a leaky blood/brain barrier into the brain. Hypothyroidism can activate brain inflammation and lead to an imbalance of the neurotransmitters. Gluten sensitivity is also an important cause of depression through the inflammatory connection, but few physicians recognize the full impact of this.

Tests for depression

There are no laboratory tests that would define depression. However, every patient should be checked for hypothyroidism, which can be a common cause of depression. If hypothyroidism is found, this can easily be treated by thyroid hormone replacement.

Otherwise the diagnosis of depression is made based on mental status examination, history and review of symptoms. A good start is to ask: "In the past 2 weeks how little interest or pleasure in doing things have you had?" and "Have you been feeling down, depressed, or hopeless in the past 2 weeks?" (Ref.3).

There are detailed psychometric questionnaires available such as the Beck Depression Inventory that can assist the physician to establish the diagnosis (1).

Myths of depression

One of the myths regarding depression is that it would be contagious (2).

A study on 2000 high school students showed that depression was not contagious like and infectious disease (3).

The contrary was true: human interaction with friends who had a "healthy mood" improved depression. By the same token, when you constantly compare yourself with your Facebook friends, and you are not in the best mood, your mood may worsen and you could become depressed.

Treatment of depression

Despite advances in the treatment of depression the response rate with antidepressant therapy is limited to 60% to 70%. According to Ref.4 inadequate dosing and misdiagnoses account for the fact that 30% to 40% of treated people with depression have treatment failures. Typically the first antidepressant involves an SSRI or selective serotonin reuptake inhibitor (4).

But newer trials have shown that the oldermonoamine oxidase inhibitors (MAOIs) have a higher success rate when treating depression initially (5).

A good antidepressant for mild to moderate depression is St. John's Wort, which is recommended by Ref. 5 as having fewer side effects as other antidepressants (6).

In treatment resistant depression the psychiatrist often employs other combinations of antidepressants. In addition cognitive/behavioral therapy is added, which makes the overall treatment more successful. It goes without saying that complicated cases of depression belong into the hands of an experienced psychiatrist.

Suicide

Unfortunately there is still a stigma attached to mental disease like depression, and people are in deep denial. Friends who do not understand depression may inadvertently say things that make the symptoms of the depressed person more severe and distance themselves at a time when they would need support from friends. The end result is loneliness, feelings of being misunderstood and having suicidal thoughts. Often it is men who will resist seeking treatment for depression; women are better in getting treatment started.

This is where a psychiatrist needs to intervene. If this does not happen, people may make suicide attempts and finally manage to commit suicide. In the US committed suicides have a gender ratio of male to female of 3:1 to 10:1 (7).

These situations become very difficult. The family needs to step in and talk to the patient. It is best to accompany the patient to the hospital for an assessment. Going to the hospital may be done privately or by ambulance. Don't be shy to call 911 for an ambulance. Better to be cautious than have a major crisis that ends in suicide.

Alternative depression treatments

There are alternative treatments for depression.
1. Magnetic therapy for depression: This therapy is also called transcranial magnetic stimulation (TMS) and was approved for Canada and in2008 by the FDA (8).

But it is not as powerful according to Ref. 3 as unitemporal electroconvulsive therapy.

2. Bifrontal electroconvulsive therapy (ECT):

Electroconvulsive therapy with two pedals applied to the front of the skull appears to have the best results in terms of treating depression (9).

3. Omega-3 fatty acids (EPA and DHA) are powerful anti-inflammatory agents, which will take care of the inflammatory component of depression. Both fish oil and krill oil in combination give the optimal response.

4. Vitamin D3 is also anti-inflammatory and will contribute to an improvement with existing depression, but it also helps prevent the development of depression when taken in regularly as a supplement.

5. Light box therapy: The observation of seasonal affective disorder (SADS) can develop as a result of lack of light. This has led to the discovery that light boxes are helpful for treating depression and also for prevention of depression due to seasonal affective disorder. A light box should be used for 30 minutes every morning during the fall and winter months. The box should emit at least 10,000 lux. Improvement can occur within 2 to 4 days of starting light therapy, but often it takes up to 4 weeks to reach its full benefit.

6. It is known for a long time that alcohol is a depressant; it can actually cause depression and in persons with bipolar disease it can trigger a flare-up of that disorder as well.

7. Finally it matters what you eat: sugar and too much starchy foods (high glycemic index carbs) lead to insulin overproduction and insulin resistance. This causes inflammation, and this will cause depression. As mentioned earlier it also lowers the two key brain transmitters, dopamine and serotonin.

The solution is an anti-inflammatory diet, the Mediterranean diet without sugar and high glycemic index carbs; only low glycemic index carbs are allowed. This will normalize insulin production and also eliminates inflammation.

8. Vitamin supplements: Folate and vitamin B12: Up to 1/3 of depressed people have folate deficiency. Supplementation with 400 mcg to 1 mg of folic acid is recommended. Vitamin B12 should also be taken to not mask a B12 deficiency (Ref.5). Folate and vitamin B12 are methyl donors for several brain neuropeptides.

9. Electro acupuncture has been shown in many studies to be effective in improving the symptoms of depression, and it seems to work through the release of neurotransmitters in the brain (Ref.6).

10. Exercise on a regular basis helps to equalize the mood and seems to exert a slight anti-depressant effect on the person who engages in regular physical activity.

Conclusion

I have attempted to show the complexity of depression and what is known about its causes and treatment. Very likely there are several causes for depression and further research will hopefully bring more clarity to this. Treatment modalities, both conventional and unconventional, have been developed over the years by trial and error. The physician and patient need to use common sense: if a treatment is working, stick to it and use it. If it does not work, move on and try something else. More difficult cases should be referred to a psychiatrist who has the most experience with difficult to treat cases. Do not neglect lifestyle factors and alternative depression treatments as they can often help to stabilize depression significantly. We all must be vigilant about suicide risks in depressed patients and act by calling 911, if necessary, to intervene.

Book references

1. Depression, Major: Fred F. Ferri M.D., F.A.C.P., Ferri's Clinical Advisor 2016, by Elsevier, Inc.

2. Dr. Datis Kharrazian: "Why Isn't My Brain Working?" © 2013, Elephant Press, Carlsbad, CA 92011

3. Goldman-Cecil Medicine "Major depressive disorder" 2016, by Saunders, an imprint of Elsevier Inc.

4. Massachusetts General Hospital Comprehensive Clinical Psychiatry, Second Edition: Theodore A. Stern MD, Maurizio Fava MD, Timothy E. Wilens MD and Jerrold F. Rosenbaum MD © 2016, Elsevier Inc.

5. Rakel: Integrative Medicine, 3rd ed. © 2012 Saunders.

6. George A. Ulett, M.D., Ph.D. and SongPing Han, B.M., Ph.D.: "The Biology of Acupuncture", copyright 2002, Warren H. Green Inc., Saint Louis, Missouri, 63132 USA

Internet references

1. http://aac.ncat.edu/newsnotes/y98fall.html
2. http://blackdoctor.org/453413/mental-illness-contagious/
3. http://articles.mercola.com/sites/articles/archive/2015/09/03/friendship-fights-depression.aspx
4. https://en.wikipedia.org/wiki/Selective_serotonin_reuptake_inhibitor
5. https://en.wikipedia.org/wiki/Monoamine_oxidase_inhibitor
6. https://en.wikipedia.org/wiki/Hypericum_perforatum

7. https://en.wikipedia.org/wiki/Gender_differences_in_suicide#United_States
8. http://www.medpagetoday.com/ProductAlert/DevicesandVaccines/11271
9. https://www.ncbi.nlm.nih.gov/pmc/articles/PMC3195158/

Publications of medical questions and answers in popular magazines.

Forbes.com: May 23, 2017

How Do Hormones Affect Emotions?

Answer by Ray Schilling, M.D., author of "Healing Gone Wrong, Healing Done Right".

1. Serotonin production in the brain is important in preventing depression. Datis Kharrazian's book "Why Isn't My Brain Working?" offers several scenarios that can cause depression and he has examples of cases that were cured of depression. He points out that deficiencies in two major brain transmitters can cause depression: serotonin and dopamine.

Serotonin is produced in the midbrain from the amino acid tryptophan in two biochemical steps. These biochemical conversions require iron, vitamin B6, vitamin B12, niacin, folic acid and magnesium as co-factors. But you also need the "large neutral amino acid transporter" (LNAA) to transport tryptophan through the blood/brain barrier into the brain.

Dopamine is a neurotransmitter that is produced in the frontal lobes of the brain. It is also necessary for learning. Dopamine is synthetized by the brain from tyrosine, which has to be manufactured in the liver from the amino acid phenylalanine. You need to have a healthy liver to produce tyrosine, which needs to be transported through the blood/brain barrier into the brain; similar to tryptophan this requires the "large neutral amino acid transporter" (LNAA). People with hepatitis, fatty liver, insulin resistance or diabetes may have problems with the LNAA transporter, which can cause dopamine deficiency. But as mentioned earlier they may also have low serotonin because tryptophan was not transported into the brain. This will happen with sugar overconsumption, as insulin resistance develops and affects the LNAA transporter resulting in both low serotonin and dopamine.

2. When testosterone is missing in an aging man, this causes low energy, depression, a lack of sex drive, and erectile dysfunction. You replace testosterone in appropriate doses and all of that normalizes. The reason for that is that many key organs, including the brain, have testosterone receptors. They need to be activated regularly by testosterone for normal organ function. Women need a small amount of testosterone as well to feel normal.

3. Estrogen hormones are the female hormones. If they are normal and balanced by progesterone (from the corpus luteum in the second half of the menstrual cycle) a woman feels well. There is a condition called estrogen dominance where too much estrogen is circulating in relation to progesterone, and these women have the following symptoms:

- Irregular or otherwise abnormal menstrual periods
- Decreased sex drive
- Bloating (water retention)
- Breast swelling and tenderness
- Fibrocystic breasts.
- Headaches (especially premenstrually)

• **Mood swings (most often irritability and depression)**

If the ratio can be normalized between progesterone and estrogen by the use of bioidentical progesterone, these symptoms disappear and the woman feels normal. Again it is the stimulation of the hormone receptors in just the right manner, which stabilizes the mood and leads to normal body function.

4. If thyroid hormones are missing, the person gets depressed and has a lack of energy. Thyroid hormones are stimulating cell function in all the body cells including the brain. Again this is transmitted by hormone receptors in the cells. It is easy for a physician to measure thyroid hormone levels (TSH and thyroid hormone levels) and to rectify the situation by ordering the right amount of thyroid hormones. When thyroid hormone receptor stimulation is normalized, all of the symptoms disappear and the person will feel normal again.

Conclusion

Hormones do not act in isolation, but in concert. Thyroid hormones give the body cells energy. Other hormones add to this and at the end we feel normal.

Chapter 14:

Detoxification

Does the skin help in detoxifying the body?

The detoxification organs are skin, kidneys and liver. Some people in the anti-aging community say that as much as 30% of the whole detoxification would be taking place in the skin. But I have not seen scientific approaches of measuring the percentage of each of the detoxification organs.

An interesting observation is the fact, that when a person eats a lot of sulfur-containing foods, any silver jewelry will turn black where the skin touches it. This is a sign that the skin can eliminate various substances, in this case sulfur compounds. It is very logical that the skin is called the largest organ of the human body!

Chapter 15:

Diabetes

Will a 600 Calorie diet help diabetes control?

The experiment has been done in Great Britain. A March 2016 study from Great Britain showed that a very-low-calorie diet for 2 months followed by a weight maintenance diet for 6 months could make diabetes reversible through diet.

Internet Reference

https://www.ncbi.nlm.nih.gov/pubmed/27002059

A total of 30 overweight or obese diabetes patients went on an 8-week very-low-calorie diet of 600-700 calories per day. 12 of these patients, the responders to this dietary approach, achieved a blood glucose level of less than 7 mmol/L (< 126 mg/dL) and an average weight loss of 14.2 kg. The others were non-responders. The responders kept their weight stable for 6 months of observation. The HbA1C fell from 7.1% to 5.8% in responders and from 8.4 to 8.0 in non-responders. The final result was that 40% of the patients got cured of diabetes.

Discussion: What this experiment shows us is that in 8 weeks 14.2 kg (=31 lbs.) was lost, that is 1.78 kg (=3.9 lbs.) per week. Not everybody was on 600 calories; some patients consumed 700 calories. In conclusion, going on a strict regimen of 600 calories per day would likely make you lose about 4.5 pounds per week.

The subjects in this experiment were all overweight or obese, and this experiment worked. If you are having a very low body weight, you should not even experiment with this restrictive diet. Anorexia would kill you! I suggest you discuss any diet plans with your physician, especially if the 600 calorie diet is involved.

Is chicken and mutton OK to eat for diabetics?

In diabetics there is a relative lack of insulin, either through insulin resistance or because of insufficient production of insulin in the pancreas.

Insulin regulates fatty acid uptake and glucose uptake. Chicken and mutton are less insulin dependent foods, and if the diabetic eats smaller portions of these meats, it will be OK to eat. Meat is broken down by digestion into amino acids, which are metabolically neutral for a diabetic.

As diabetes is an inflammatory disease, it is best to adopt an anti inflammatory diet like the DASH diet or the Mediterranean diet. These diets have a solid track record of being very useful to treat diabetics. In these diets there is an emphasis on vegetables, salads, whole grains in small amounts, lean meats and fish.

Chapter 16:

Diet

I want to get rid of sugar in my diet. How can I do this long-term?

1. In February of 2001 my wife and I attended an anti-aging conference in San Diego. The keynote speaker was Dr. Barry Sears who is the inventor of the zone diet (1). We had read a book from him before the conference and were excited to hear him speak in person. We liked the book; we liked the talk, so we cut out sugar, starchy foods and stuck to a diet where the calories derived 50% from low-glycemic, complex carbohydrates, 25-30% from lean meat, poultry and fish. Calories derived from fat were reduced to about 15-20% (there is hidden fat even in lean meat). No butter, but instead some cheeses with low to medium fat contents and olive oil for cooking and in salad dressings. We both lost 50 pounds each! That's a lot of weight. All our clothes had to be brought to the tailor to make them fit again.

2. Before we started to cut out sugar and starchy foods, we went though the contents of our fridge and looked at all of the labels on the various products. One third of the content had to be thrown out, as it was incompatible with

a sensible diet. Not adding any additional sugar was easy, but things like jams that have 45% to 50% of sugar in them had to be removed as well. Bread had to go, soft drinks (=sugary drinks) had no place any more. It was quite an eye opener.

3. We acquired body composition scales, which give information about fat percentage including visceral fat percentage, muscle mass percentage, BMI, weight and the basic metabolic rate. We wanted to define the end point of what our ideal body weight would be. We are avid ballroom and Latin dancers, but we noticed that our dance program was not good enough to lower the BMI below about 23.5; using the body composition scales we noted that our body fat content was still too high and the visceral fat percentage was still in the 6% range (2). It took a prolonged trip to the US where we could not find enough dance events to decide that we would introduce a one hour gym program consisting of 30 minutes of treadmill, 15 minutes of upper body circuits, and 15 minutes of lower body circuits every day as a basis to our exercise program. Any dance activity would be just an additional exercise on top of the base exercise from the gym (3). It took only about 2 months before our fat composition decreased, our muscle mass increased, the visceral fat went to a normal at 5% and the BMI was now stabilized at the 21.5 to 22.0 range.

4. Maintenance of our no sugar program: In the meantime we shop at the periphery of a grocery store:

Let's start at the deli: your low fat cheese varieties, roasted chicken or turkey breast or lean ham if you choose are all found here.

Go on to the meats: lean cuts of beef, pork, chicken, lamb will be found here, and next will be
Fish and seafood: salmon, sole, cod, halibut, trout, mussels, shrimp will be there to choose from.

Continue at the vegetarian section: tofu, tempeh, and vegetarian burgers, low fat cottage cheese, and more low fat variety of cheeses.

The bakery section is also found at the periphery, but you will want to be very discerning. Most of the selection is not offering more than highly refined carbohydrates and trans fats. The dozen bagels will not offer you much nutritional bang for your buck!

Finally you will arrive at the produce department. You will likely go for all the green leaf choices like leaf lettuce, kale, chard, spinach, as well as the cabbage varieties (broccoli, green cabbage, sui choy, napa cabbage, cauliflower).

The other ones of your list are the intensely colored non-root vegetables like tomatoes, red and green peppers, also mushrooms, which are a power house of minerals, green beans, asparagus, as well as onions and garlic. You will also buy your fruit: apples, oranges, grapefruit and other citrus, pears, berries, and pineapple. You will go easy on mango, papaya and banana because of their high sugar content.

The deep frozen section can be your best ally: look for deep frozen vegetables, fruit, and fish as well as meats. As vegetables are quickly readied for the freezer, their vitamin content can be higher than that of a vegetable that has spent 8 days in transit from the field to the produce department. The deep frozen section also gives you access to a lot of variety. You'll be able to enjoy some strawberries, even when they are not in season. Read the labels, as some fruit have been packaged with sugar syrup. Look for the varieties, where no sugar has been added. The frozen section also contains some highly processed items: deep-fried foods and dessert selections, which may not be an accessory to full health but rather to an empty wallet.

Canned foods can be useful, as long as you are dealing with fruit that are canned in their juices and not in sugar syrup. The vegetables are less valuable in vitamins than their deep frozen counterparts. Watch out for varieties, where less salt is added. The label will tell you "low sodium".

You will not have to navigate all the aisles, except for your cleaning products and your cosmetics. There are some staples, which you will also require: olive oil, some olives, almonds or macadamia nuts (raw or dry roasted). The one cereal product, which is valuable, will be coarse rolled oats and some pot barley. Both varieties carry a lot of fibre, which makes them very useful food staples. Avoid the "quick cooking" or "instant" oats. Due to the processing, the carbohydrates are absorbed a lot faster and consequently trigger a higher insulin response.

You'll wonder about drinks next. Having passed the colas, ginger ales and other sugar pops you may eye the diet drinks. Beware of drinks sweetened with aspartame. There is increasing evidence that phenylalanine (brand names: Aspartame, NutraSweet and Sweet'N Low) is not a "harmless" sweetener. Newer research has shown that it can cause gastroesophageal reflux (=GERD) and migraine headaches. Stevia, a sweetener from a South American plant, does not have harmful effects, and stevia, which is safe to use, as it does not cause an insulin response. You are best served with mineral water, purified drinking water, herb teas, tea or coffee. Fruit juices do have vitamins and minerals, but they are high in sugar causing an insulin release.

You would not really eat 3 large apples in one sitting. So why insist on drinking 8 oz. of apple juice? You'll ingest all the sugar and forgo the fibre! You'll also notice that a lot of fruit juices have been mixed with sugar, water, artificial flavor, some color, and as an apology some vitamin C has been added. They are appearing on the shelves as "a good source of vitamin C". In reality we are dealing with flavoured, colorful sugar water. Use your own judgement, whether you want to spend your dollars on this selection! In the aisle adjacent to the pop you will very likely encounter a huge selection of convenience and snack foods. They have several things in common: you have met them on TV, some will be high in starches and fat (chips), others will be high in starches, sugar, and fat (cookies, donuts, cream pastries), and we are dealing with trans fats. Do take time to read the listed ingredients, and then decide, whether you and those who eat in your household deserve nutritional garbage.

You have now completed your round trip in the supermarket.

To sum up the most important facts, remember the following:

- Do most of your shopping at the periphery of the store.
- Look for fresh products – the less processed, the better.
- Read the ingredients on labels.
- Stay away from nutritional garbage

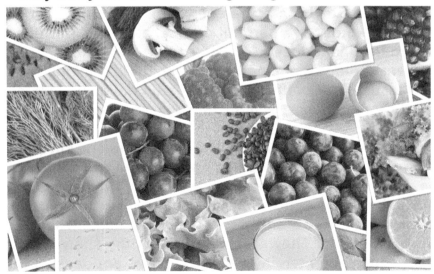

Internet references

1. https://www.drsears.com/
2. https://en.wikipedia.org/wiki/Adipose_tissue
3. https://www.wikihow.com/Get-Fit-in-the-Gym

What would happen, if I removed all sugar except fruit and honey from my diet?

That's what I did in 2001. But I also cut out honey, as this is identical to sugar. The reason that is important is that sugar raises LDL cholesterol and triglycerides and causes heart attacks and strokes. In the prior answered question I explained in detail how my wife and I have done this. We both lost 50 pounds each.

But I like my coffee sweet, so I use a tiny bit of stevia, a natural sweetener. It is harder to only partially eliminate sugar (if you continue to eat honey), than to go all the way and reward yourself by non-sugar sweetening. But don't fall into the trap of other sweeteners that are dangerous. Sucralose is particularly bad, as it actually is a by-product of insecticide research remarketed as "useful sweetener" for diabetics.

To answer your question "What would happen, if I removed all sugar except fruit from my diet?" The answer is "nothing": you just will lose weight until you reach your ideal body weight. During the initial days of eliminating sugar, you may feel a sense of withdrawal. Some people get grumpy or complain of a headache. If you have these symptoms, do not give up! The health benefits of eliminating sugar are numerous and all worth it: normal weight, less heart disease, less inflammation, less arthritis.

Publications of medical questions and answers in popular magazines.

forbes.com: Oct. 11, 2017

How Do Our Bodies Use Carbohydrates?

Answer by Ray Schilling, M.D., author of "Healing Gone Wrong, Healing Done Right".

    Carbs are varied. There are complex carbohydrates that are absorbed slowly and you hardly get an insulin reaction. On the other end of the spectrum there are refined carbs like sugar, which are rapidly absorbed in the gut and to which the body reacts swiftly with an insulin reaction to lower high blood sugars.
    Generally speaking, all carbs are broken down into glucose and absorbed in the gut. Glucose is the fuel that is metabolized inside the cells in the mitochondria to give us energy (1).
    This is particularly important in the brain, which lives solely by glucose as the energy supply, but our muscles, our heart, our liver and kidneys are all very rich in mitochondria for the metabolism of glucose.
    There is a dark side to refined carbs that we need to know about: when all our glucose storage spaces in the liver and the muscles are full (glycogen is the storage form of glucose), then the liver starts processing glucose. With our sugar consumption having spiralled upwards in the last 183 years, this surplus sugar metabolism is causing more and more problems.
    The liver produces triglycerides from the extra sugar and LDL cholesterol, the bad cholesterol. This causes the hardening of arteries and causes heart attacks, strokes and high blood pressure.

We need to come to our senses and cut out processed foods (which has extra sugar in it), switch to a Mediterranean diet and only consume complex carbs, contained in legumes, vegetables and fruit. It is also recommendable to cut out starchy foods with a glycemic index of higher than 55 in order to bring our liver metabolism back to normal (normal triglyceride and LDL cholesterol production). This will mean cutting out pasta, potatoes, rice, bread and muffins.

Internet reference

1. https://www.ncbi.nlm.nih.gov/books/NBK9896/

Is there one particular food component that makes us fat and obese?

I think that this is a reasonable question to ask. The one foodstuff that was not present 150 years ago was refined sugar. Not only is it available as a substance on many tables around coffee time, but it also is mixed into many foods like yogurt, jams, cereals, bakery products, power bars etc.

So, here is a review of what it does to your body.

You need to understand that starchy foods equal sugar, once digested. As a result a refined cereal breakfast equals sugar, pasta is converted into sugar and that slice of bread- especially a toast from white bread is converted into sugar. You can continue the list with donuts, potatoes and white rice, and so on. It has to do with the glycemic load (1). When you cut out sugar and starchy foods (meaning that the glycemic index of the foods you eat is below 50) you will shed 30 to 50 pounds of weight within 3 to 5 months, if you are overweight or obese. You will feel a lot more energy. Your blood vessels will be cleaned out as the oxidized LDL cholesterol will disappear and the HDL cholesterol will mop up what cholesterol deposits were there before.

It is certainly good for you, if you are not into the sugar and candy stuff, but the seemingly harmless pizza and all the other starchy foods mentioned above are of concern as well. All of the high-glycemic carbs stimulate the pancreas to produce insulin. This in turn produces inflammation in tissues, including the brain. Alzheimer's disease is one of the complications of this.

Where does this leave us? For decades we have been told that saturated fats and cholesterol in our diet were the culprits, and we replaced them with sugar that is part of a low-fat diet. We need to pay attention to the glycemic index and cut out high glycemic foods.

However, it is OK to eat some carbs from the medium glycemic food list and most of our carbs from the low glycemic food list. With regard to fat it is important to consume only the healthy fats like olive oil, coconut oil and omega-3 fatty acids. As you make these adjustments to your life style you will also prevent many cancers, as you normalize the body's metabolism and help prevent chronic inflammation, which can cause arthritis and cancer. Finally, pay attention to stress management. The body and the mind work together. Uncontrolled stress can also lead to heart attacks and strokes.

Internet reference

1. http://lpi.oregonstate.edu/mic/food-beverages/glycemic-index-glycemic-load

Can you live for 4 years on only microwave cooked food?

From the way this question was written, it seems that there is the notion that "microwave cooking is bad for you". This is a myth and has not been scientifically proven. Instead it has been proven that microwave cooking preserves vitamins better than regular cooking on a stove, as the process is faster (1).

Here is the answer: eating microwave oven cooked food for four years is not any different than regularly oven cooked food, except microwaved food may have retained a few more vitamins.

Internet reference

1. https://cnneatocracy.wordpress.com/2014/01/22/does-microwaving-nuke-nutrition/

Why do dieticians often support nutritional principles that are miles apart, for instance Vegan versus Paleo versus Mediterranean diets?

This is an interesting question. It is true that nutritional gurus have recommended diets that are totally opposite for a long time.

1. For instance the low fat/high carb diet has ruled for over 30 years. It was thought that saturated fats would have been the cause of elevated cholesterol. But later it turned out that it was high carbs that caused high LDL cholesterol, fat deposits from sugar being metabolized in the liver into fatty substances and subsequently being deposited as fat. Finally the low fat/high carb diet was identified as the cause of the obesity wave and is now officially abandoned.

2. This is now replaced by the Mediterranean diet, which is a low carb/medium healthy fat diet. This is an anti-inflammatory diet that is balanced, but avoids sugar and high-glycemic, starchy foods (avoiding high-glycemic carbs).

3. Here is another example: Dr. Steven Masley and Dr. Jonny Bowden wrote a book recently: "Smart Fat. Eat more fat. Lose more weight. Get Healthy now". (Harper One, 2016, New York). In the beginning they explain that both came from extreme diet backgrounds and they met in the middle, now publishing this book. Dr. Masley, a cardiologist, was a director of the Pritikin Longevity Center for many years. The Pritikin diet is an ultra-low-fat eating plan with whole, unprocessed foods high in fiber and complex carbohydrates. Dr. Bowden, a nutritionist supported the ultra-low-carb, high protein Atkins diet. Both made the observation that after a few months or years, people could not stand their diets any more, and they regained their weight as they returned to their previous bad diet habits. In this book they proclaim a middle of the road diet with healthy fats, a lot of fiber and the right amount of clean protein (meat from grass-fed animals or organic meats).

I have poor eating habits and also bad sleeping habits. Does that affect my health?

1. First to the abnormal sleeping pattern: You are deliberately going against your built-in hormones. The reason we make cortisol in the adrenal glands is that we are be ready for the fight/flight response during the day and cope with stress naturally. You seem to be awake most of the night, which prevents you from getting melatonin that would put you to sleep, because in the presence of artificial light, the pineal gland does not release melatonin. Your body makes melatonin and stores it in your pineal

gland, but your behaviour prevents you from benefiting from melatonin. With your sleep pattern you are missing the midnight to 3 AM human growth hormone peak. Your brain releases that hormone only during your deepest sleep and only between midnight and 3 AM.

2. Irregular meals: Your body receives breakfast at 4 AM. Then you skip breakfast, because your stomach is already full. You sleep from 10 AM to 2 PM. Of course, you will often miss lunch, because you are sleeping. Dinner seems to be light and maybe at a normal time? The problem with these off-time meals is that your body needs energy all of the time. I suspect that you are also snacking, and it may not be the healthiest food. When you go for long periods without a meal you become hypoglycemic and suddenly turn very hungry, which usually translates into reaching for unhealthy snacks. This is how many people gain weight (sugar/fat snacks).

3. Here is what I recommend:

a) Go to bed between 10 PM and 11 PM. Sleep for 7 to 8 hours. When you do, you will make human growth hormone again, which is needed for your daytime energy. This way you won't need any sleep until bedtime at 10 PM. You were human growth hormone deficient and that's why you needed daytime naps to rebuild your energy. With regular sleep habits you will have energy all day long.

b) Eat three meals a day, breakfast, lunch and dinner. Follow a Mediterranean diet. Cut out sugar and starchy foods. Have lots of vegetables, fruit, nuts, seafood, lean chicken and turkey. If you want to eat beef, make sure it is grass-fed beef, and eat it only once per week. Bison is better than beef.

4. You asked what health consequences your behavior may have. Your irregular sleeping habit interferes with your hormone system: human growth hormone low, melatonin suboptimal, cortisol too much; sex hormones too low (not

enough nighttime sleep). You will also be more susceptible for reactive hypoglycemia from insulin overproduction, which causes craving for unhealthy sugary foods. On the long term you may be susceptible to high blood pressure, gaining weight from unhealthy snacks and diabetes. The question is whether you eat healthy food with healthy bacteria in it to take care of your gut bacteria. It is very important to take probiotics. You can get this from the health food store. Stay away from wheat and wheat products in processed foods. It contains a lot of gliadin, which creates leaky gut syndrome. Once you establish that you get autoantibodies. This can cause arthritis and many other illnesses. Chronic inflammation can also cause high blood pressure, heart attacks and strokes as well as type-2 diabetes. It is much better to prevent all this than get into this downward spiral of deteriorating health.

Going to bed late has consequences. I summarized this under this question, the answer to which you find under "Sleep": "What happens when you go to bed late every night?"

Why do some Americans prefer processed, preserved or packaged foods to farm-fresh food?

It started in the 1950's and 1960's when American firms realized that they could make it easy for the consumer to have pre-packaged dinners (TV dinners). Then fast food chains developed like McDonald's and others. Chinese take-out orders joined the club, and pizza to take out became fashionable. The mid section of the grocery store became bigger and bigger while the vegetable and deli section stayed about the same in size in the periphery except for the dairy section. Sugar laden yogurt and yogurt drinks were and still are selling fiercely. The reason? It's convenient. You do not have to do anything except open a lid and you can start to eat.

In the meantime Americans are used to these packaged food items. Many do not even read the ingredients. They just trust the food companies that the food will be "healthy".

Back in 2001 my wife and I read every food label of any food item we bought. We came to the conclusion that there is more junk in the middle section of a grocery store than we ever thought possible. Mostly it is sugar content, but salt content is too high also, and various food chemicals and preservatives are in pre-packaged foods that you do not want to eat.

As a result we simplified our food list and avoid as much of the pre-packaged items as possible. We like to buy whole foods and prepare our meals ourselves. We avoid sugar (we don't buy it). Instead we use stevia, a natural plant sweetener. Most of our food is organic.

We don't eat processed meat. We eat little meat, and moderate amounts of fish (wild salmon).

The answer to your question is that many Americans find it more convenient to eat processed foods, but they are trading it in for a lack of quality.

Are fruit unhealthy due to their sugar content?

The answer is "no". But the better question to ask is: is sugar from fruit better for you than white sugar. And the answer is "yes" (1).

As the link explains sugar in fruit is bound to fiber, which releases sugar more slowly. Sugar is sucrose, a disaccharide with one molecule of fructose bound to one molecule of glucose. When we digest a meal with sugar in it, the enzyme sucrose splits sugar into fructose and glucose sucrose. Both are taken up into the bloodstream. The liver processes fructose, glucose enters our body cells directly with the help of insulin.

If we eat the fruit unprocessed, the sugar in them is healthy, because the fiber keeps it bound for some time and the body has time to process some of the released sugar as it is digested. If we eat too much dried fruit (raisins, dried cherries etc.) or white sugar from candies or cakes the sugar reaches unhealthy heights in the blood, an enormous insulin response, and the liver produces high amounts of triglycerides and LDL cholesterol. This leads to hardening of the arteries, heart attacks and strokes.

I have replaced all added sugar by stevia, a plant based sweetener. I do not use processed food with sugar in it (I always read food labels). Eating vegetables and fruit keeps me away from high sugar concentrations.

Internet reference

1. http://www.huffingtonpost.com/2013/06/29/fruit-sugar-versus-white-sugar_n_3497795.html

Is there a difference between cheap and expensive chocolate?

Sugar is cheap and cocoa is expensive. Most chocolate manufacturers want to sell you a sugar-laden chocolate product, but what you are really getting is candy. The healthy bioflavonoids are contained in the cocoa part of chocolate. I don't buy anything less than 80% cocoa content chocolate. But there is still too much sugar in this chocolate!

I got tired of compromising having to eat sugar, when I want to eat a chocolate. My wife and I perfected making our own chocolate:

You may wonder how we solved the dark chocolate problem, which by the way would double as a gluten-free food: You buy 100 % unsweetened Baker's chocolate or 100% Ghirardelli chocolate (0 g sugar on the label) and liquefy it in a little bowl in a pot with hot water. Add a tiny bit of stevia sweetener and add a tiny bit of vanilla extract into the well-stirred chocolate liquid. Prepare a form out of aluminum foil with a rim or else use a small square plastic container into which you carefully pour the content (watch it, hot!) and let it sit to cool down. When it is at room temperature, cut into smaller pieces, which you keep in a glass jar in the fridge. This is 100% gluten-free chocolate, 100% chocolate and 100% healthy. This will not get you addicted, as chocolate itself is not addicting, it is the sugar that's addicting.

This chocolate is not inexpensive as I said in the beginning: cocoa is expensive and sugar is cheap.

Some foods are advertised healthy, but they are actually not?

One example is Stevia Coke. It is heavily advertised as a lower calorie soft drink. Stevia by itself would have no calories and is an excellent natural sweetener. But when you read the label, it contains 25 grams of sugar per small bottle. This is the equivalent of 5 teaspoons of sugar. This shows you how powerful the sugar industry is and how deceptive big companies are with their false advertising! Strangely enough, there is a line of soft drinks, Zevia that only has stevia-sweetened drinks.

Why is that important? Sugar causes hardening of arteries because it is metabolized in the liver and causes high LDL cholesterol and high triglycerides. These fatty substances end up in the lining of the arteries and fat gets deposited in subcutaneous fatty tissue with the help of insulin. The end result: heart attacks and strokes. There are also more deaths, and it is not healthy. That's why I decided to cut out sugar and sugar in processed foods.

What is the difference between regular and steel-cut oats?

Oats grow as a grain. Oats come in three basic forms.

1. Regular or fast oats where the bran has been taken out and you can instantly eat them by adding milk or water to them. When you buy them (DON'T !), they look like small little flakes in the package. Because the FIBER HAS BEEN TAKEN OUT, do not eat these: they bring your LDL cholesterol up and eventually raise your triglycerides as well, which will cause heart attacks and strokes on the long term. It is a carbohydrate which has been refined, and your body will convert it into sugar.

2. Rolled oats or old-fashioned oats: they are my favorites. They were steamed and rolled in the factory, but they left the bran in them. They look like big flakes in the package when you buy them. For people with gluten sensitivity there are gluten free rolled oats available in health food stores. Rolled oats are ready for use, even if they are not cooked. Because they had been precooked in the factory they will taste good when you add liquid (yogurt, goat milk or organic milk) to them, fruit, a bit of cinnamon and a tiny bit of stevia to sweeten (NO SUGAR). Why no sugar, you ask? Because this will raise your LDL cholesterol and triglycerides over time and cause heart attacks and strokes, the very thing you want to prevent by having a healthy breakfast. But, if you prepare it the way I described, you will lower LDL cholesterol and triglycerides and you prevent heart attacks and strokes. When your grandmother told you to eat oats, she meant the old fashioned rolled oats.

3. Steel-cut oats. This product is newer in North America, but has been around for a long time in Scotland and Ireland. I think we are coming closer to your question: a

steel cutter, which made smaller pieces out of the oat grain, cut steel-cut oats. This almost looks more like birdseeds, but is more irregular. Steel-cut oats are still raw grains. You would not enjoy eating them right away, as they can't be digested easily. In order to make them digestible you have to put them into a slow cooker together with enough water overnight, so they are ready to eat in the morning. Alternatively, if you forgot to prepare them overnight, you have to cook them in water for 25 minutes before you are ready to do the other preparations for breakfast. I don't know about you. But I do not want to take that time. That's why option 2 is my choice. The good news: yes, the bran is still in steel-cut oats and you will lower LDL cholesterol and triglycerides, so no heart attacks and strokes.

Oats are an exceptional food. They are perfect for a quick breakfast and are also easy to take along when you travel.

Too much refined sugar can make you sick. Is it as bad as cigarettes?

The following will show you that sugar actually is as bad as cigarettes for you. The key is to avoid both.

It has been known for a long time that cancer cells can survive without the ordinary aerobic pathways of energy production. They can get energy from a metabolic pathway, which bypasses normal cell metabolism, called aerobic glycolysis (1).

But many attempts of designing a cancer therapy to exploit this difference have so far been unsuccessful.

This Mayo Clinic website even explains that it would be a myth that cancer would grow better with sugar (2).

The following pieces of research question this myth.

Sugar makes cancer grow faster (activates oncogenes) in fruit flies

In this study from the Icahn School of Medicine at Mount Sinai in New York City fruit flies were used as an animal model. You may ask, why fruit flies? But we are not fruit flies, we are humans! As incredible as it sounds, on a cellular level our cell metabolism and the cell metabolism of fruit flies is identical. But the generation time of fruit flies is much shorter and results can be seen in days and weeks. To achieve the same in human trials would take months and years. Also, researchers could breed a strain of fruit flies that was susceptible to develop tumors. When they were fed sugar, the fruit flies developed insulin resistance within a short time. This model was chosen by the researchers as it is known for some time that in human insulin resistance from diabetes, obesity, and other metabolic diseases leads to a higher risk of developing breast cancer, liver cancer, colon cancer and pancreatic cancer. The researchers wanted to sort out what the metabolic advantage of the cancer cells was under these conditions.

The researchers found that the sugar in the diet activated silent cancer causing genes (called "oncogenes") in the fruit flies that in turn helped to promote insulin resistance and the development of tumors. Because of the insulin resistance sugar could not enter into the normal body cells, but the tumor was using up all of the sugar allowing the tumor cells to multiply at a rapid rate. The end result was that the sugar from the diet fed the cancer cells directly making them grow faster. Interestingly, when these flies that had developed tumors on a high sugar diet were switched to a high protein/low sugar diet, the tumors stopped growing and were contained.

In this fruit fly example the researchers were subsequently able to block cancer cell growth by special cancer suppressing drugs (acarbose, pyrvinium and an experimental drug AD81), which were given in combination. 90% of the flies given the triple-drug treatment survived to adulthood while control flies not treated with this regimen all died of their tumors.

Although this model was only done in fruit flies and one could question whether or not this was relevant to what is happening in human cancer patients, the following piece of research puts this fear to rest.

Human breast cancer cell study in vitro

In January 2014 the American Society for Clinical Investigation published a collaborative study between the Lawrence Berkeley National Laboratory, Berkeley, California, CA and the Hokkaido University Graduate School of Medicine, Japan, which used human breast cells in tissue culture showing that sugar could cause breast cancer.

The original papers of this US/Japanese research team are quite technical and I do not expect you to understand this link where it is published (3). I posted it for those who want in depth information. The researchers used a simple tissue culture model where they could observe tumor growth in cell cultures under the microscope using a gel where the breast tissue samples were placed side by side with normal breast cells that served as controls (4).

The cell cultures of both normal cells and malignant cells were obtained from the same reduction mammoplasty tissue samples. This way the cell cultures mimicked a situation as close to the reality of what is going on in a woman's body when breast cancer develops.

The normal breast epithelial cells were seen in culture to get organized as a roundish cell formation, (an acinus formation), while the cancer cells were growing as irregular cell clumps. This visual effect was reproducible and is depicted in the paper (5).

With high sugar concentrations in the growth medium breast cancer cells multiplied at a faster rate, not so the normal cells. But some normal cells underwent a transformation into abnormal and cancerous cell types. On the other hand, when sugar concentrations were severely restricted, morphological changes took place where cancer cells slowed down their growth or stagnated while some of them even changed into the normal cell formation (acinus formation). Using various known oncogene stabilizers the investigators could show that the same effect was noted as with the low sugar concentration in the growth medium.

The investigators tested whether other cell lines of breast cancer would show similar results as to the effects of sugar feeding or restriction. They were able to show that high sugar feeding activated cancer cells, no matter where the cancer cell lines originated. The authors discussed that metformin, which is known to control the metabolism in diabetic patients and lowers blood sugar levels, has also been shown to calm down growth of cancer (due to stopping oncogene stimulation), which improves the survival rates of many different cancer types in diabetic patients; it also reduces the risk of developing cancer in those who are taking metformin.

Other investigators have shown in mouse experiments that an impressive lowering of cancer rates could be achieved with low carb diets (6).

Human evidence for cancer causation and cancer prevention

Several clinical studies seem to indicate that there is a higher cancer rate in diabetics where insulin resistance can lead to activation of cancer producing genes (called oncogenes) and cause various cancers. In this link colorectal cancer and pancreatic cancer are discussed in relationship to diabetes and insulin resistance (7).

High glycemic foods (sugar and starchy foods) were associated with breast cancer, colorectal cancer and endometrial cancer (8).

The majority of trials showed this association, although not all. The more obese patients were, the more pronounced the insulin resistance was and the more the relationship to these cancers became apparent. A diet that is high in starchy foods like potatoes, rice and bread is causing pancreatic cancer as was shown by researchers at the Dana-Faber Cancer Institute, Brigham and Women's Hospital and Harvard School of Public Health (9).

High glycemic diets have shown to cause colorectal cancer, diabetes and they also cause weight gain (10).

The Standard North American Diet (SAD) is a pathway to many chronic illnesses due its high load in refined carbohydrates. Ironically the abbreviation for it is "SAD", which in my opinion reflects adequately its sad influence on health and well being. We know now that sugar and starchy foods lead to insulin overproduction, which in turn causes the metabolic syndrome (also known as "insulin resistance"). This causes the immune system to weaken and fat to be deposited as visceral fat in the stomach area. Visceral fat is metabolically very active as it secretes cytokines like tumor necrosis factor alpha (TNF alpha), COX-2 enzymes and others. Insulin and growth factors from the visceral fat gang up together with the elevated blood sugar, which activates tumor-producing genes (oncogenes) to cause cancer.

While cancer rates are higher in patients with insulin resistance, they were lower in patients who did have normal insulin levels. It is important to concentrate your efforts on normalizing weight, which will normalize insulin sensibility and avoid the development of cancer. Sugar avoidance and avoidance of refined cereals and starchy foods will help you achieve this goal.

Conclusion

Although the idea that sugar could cause cancer has been around since 1924 (Dr. Warburg), it has taken up to now to be proven in animals and humans (11).

The purpose of this outline was to show how there is a connection between the consumption of sugar and starchy foods and various cancers in man. Animal experiments are useful in suggesting these connections, but many clinical trials including the Women's Health Initiative have shown that these findings are also true in humans (12).

It is insulin resistance due to sugar and starch over-consumption that is causing cancer.

We are now in a position to know why people who consume a low carb diet, develop less cancer than people who consume a high carb diet. I have followed such a low carb diet (also known as low-glycemic index food diet) since 2001 and find it easy to follow. However, I do not dispute that it takes some discipline to change the old way of eating to the new one. The benefits are definitely worth it: you are feeling well, and you are staying well as you age.

Here is more information about hyperinsulinemia that can cause breast cancer (13).

This blog was published first on Feb. 8, 2014: "Sugar As A Cause Of Cancer" (14).

Internet references

1. https://en.wikipedia.org/wiki/Glycolysis
2. http://www.mayoclinic.org/diseases-conditions/cancer/in-depth/cancer-causes/art-20044714?pg=2

3. http://www.jci.org/articles/view/63146
4. https://www.ncbi.nlm.nih.gov/pubmed/17396127
5. http://www.jci.org/articles/view/63146/figure/3
6. https://www.sciencedaily.com/releases/2011/06/110614115037.htm
7. https://academic.oup.com/jnci/article/92/3/192/2965027/Diabetes-and-Cancer-Scientists-Search-for-a
8. http://lpi.oregonstate.edu/mic/food-beverages/glycemic-index-glycemic-load
9. https://www.foodnavigator.com/Article/2002/09/05/High-starch-diet-linked-to-cancer
10. https://www.hsph.harvard.edu/nutritionsource/carbohydrates/carbohydrates-and-blood-sugar/
11. https://en.wikipedia.org/wiki/Warburg_hypothesis
12. https://en.wikipedia.org/wiki/Women%27s_Health_Initiative
13. http://nethealthbook.com/cancer-overview/breast-cancer/causes-breast-cancer/
14. http://www.askdrray.com/sugar-as-a-cause-of-cancer/

Let's assume I don't eat sugar for one year. What would happen?

If you eliminate added sugar, you will notice that your weight goes down at a rate of 1 to 2 pounds per week. It depends how much added sugar you were consuming.

You need to be aware that you likely also eat a fair amount of carbohydrates (bread, rice, noodles, muffins etc.) that turn into sugar in your gut through digestion.

If you cut out these empty calories as well you will likely lose 2 to 3 pounds per week until you get close to your ideal body weight. At that point your weight loss slows down and reaches a plateau.

The surprising part is that despite your weight loss you will feel more energetic.

Read the answer above to the following question regarding details about how you would go shopping to buy the right foods: I want to get rid of sugar in my diet. How can I do this long-term?

What are some key facts about healthy food consumption?

You want to know how to turn older, but stay healthier (no diseases, no disabilities)? Here is how to do it:

1. Cut out sugar. This prevents diabetes, heart attacks and strokes.

2. Avoid processed meats: this reduces the risk of some cancers.

3. Eat clean foods: organic vegetables or your own vegetables grown in your garden; organic salad; grass-fed beef once per week (not more often); organic chicken and turkey; bison meat once every week or every two weeks; wild salmon two to three times per week.

4. If you exercise regularly on top of eating healthy foods, you half all illnesses and diseases compared to those who don't.

5. I also cut out starchy foods as they turn into sugar and give you an insulin response causing hyperinsulinemia, inflammation in your arteries, strokes, heart attacks and Alzheimer's. If you can do it and you don't want those diseases: cut out wheat and wheat products; pasta, bread, baked goods with flour in it, potatoes, white rice and cereal. I have done this since 2001, lost 50 pounds and kept it down since. My body mass index is between 21 and 22. I have energy, work out and do all those things.

Thought experiment: take our food from today and introduce it into a medieval village in Europe. What would happen to the population?

A similar thing would happen as what did happen to the German population after WWII. The basic nutrition was simple at that time. Germans ate rye bread, but wheat was introduced more and more. The bakeries mixed wheat into rye bread and called it mixed bread ("Mischbrot"). By the early 1960's most bread was just wheat flour bread alone. Toast became something trendy. But it is utterly devoid of fiber. Fast foods came to Germany in the 1960's and even more so in the 1970's. The end result was that diabetes flourished, the first obesity wave hit Germany with millions of heart attacks and strokes. The diets of civilized countries, in the US it is called Standard American Diet (SAD), caused inflammation within the blood vessels, in the joints and the brain. The extra sugar causes tooth decay and gum disease. This is the reason why heart attacks, strokes, high blood pressure, arthritis, diabetes, Parkinson's disease, Alzheimer's disease and many more illnesses develop.

So, essentially you're asking what would have happened, if someone had introduced the SAD diet into a village or town in medieval Europe. I have no doubts that exactly the same would have happened to people then that are happening to people today. Right now we are experiencing the second obesity wave, largely because of an increased consumption of sugar, starchy foods and corn syrup. There is a diabetes wave, an Alzheimer's and Parkinson's disease wave, an arthritis wave etc. Why would this happen? Because food can change our metabolic balance as outlined below.

1. Inflammation is causing the illnesses already mentioned. Inflammation also comes from a change of

gut bacteria where the beneficial flora is replaced by undesirable bacteria. This leads to inflammation: Just How Can Bacteria Be 'Healthy' For Your Body (1)?

2. The overload with omega-6 fatty acids from processed foods, mostly from soybean oil is causing a disbalance of the omega-6 to omega-3 ratio. Fish and seafood provide you with healthy omega-3 fatty acids (2).

Unfortunately not all fish are healthy and safe to eat. Tuna is a predator fish that accumulates a lot of mercury from the polluted oceans. As a result of this it is not on my fish list. I prefer wild salmon. I also take molecularly distilled fish oil, which has omega-3 fatty acids in it. Many processed foods contain only omega-6 fatty acids, because this is the cheapest way to produce them (they are based on vegetable oils). Also, avoid soybean oil, which is the most popular oil in the last few decades to foul up the omega-6 to omega-3 ratio. This ratio should be 1:1 to 3:1, but many Americans' omega-6 to omega-3 ratio is 6:1 to 18:1. Omega-6-fatty acids cause arthritis, heart disease and strokes. Instead you want to eat healthy fats like omega-3 fatty acids contained in nuts and fish. You can also add molecularly distilled, high potency omega-3 fatty acids as a supplement to help restore the balance between omega-6 and omega-3 in your food intake.

3. Overconsumption of alcohol and red meat, the typical diet of the affluent in the past (kings included) causes gout and arthritis. It is still happening now. The elimination of alcohol in the kidneys is interfering with the breakdown of purines, causing a back up of uric acid in the blood with precipitation of uric acid crystals in and around joints, which is extremely painful. In the middle ages, royalty was suffering from gout as is amply documented in history books. King Henry VIII was one of them and was sick and miserable.

Conclusion

Modern junk food would be as effective making you sick in a medieval town in Europe as it is effective now wherever it is consumed. The key is to learn from this medieval thought experiment and use this information to prevent the deterioration of your health from a bad diet.

Internet references

1. https://www.scienceabc.com/humans/good-bad-gut-bacteria-human-body-probiotics-healthy.html
2. http://www.umm.edu/health/medical/altmed/supplement/omega3-fatty-acids/

I have eaten a lot of unhealthy food. What's the best thing I can do to become healthier now?

1. When you eat a lot of junk foods, you eat too much sugar, too much processed foods and too many refined carbs. You may also eat hydrogenated fats. The sugar and starchy food overload leads to an accumulation of fructose-1,6-bisphosphate, a metabolic by-product from sugar consumption. It stimulates a RAS gene, which can mutate, turn into an oncogene and eventually cause cancer (1).
2. What you need to do is simply to adopt a Mediterranean diet. Avoid refined sugar consumption; avoid processed foods, because they contain too much sugar. This will change insulin resistance into insulin sensitivity. Fructose-1,6-bisphosphate will not accumulate, but get normally metabolized. This way fructose-1,6-bisphosphate does not pose a problem for RAS proteins. Your insulin level will normalize, the previous kinin overproduction will disappear and your risk for cancer will decrease.

3. But this is not the only benefit of avoiding junk food. The second benefit is that you minimize, better even cut out completely your consumption of hydrogenated fats. Hydrogenated fats like margarine are considered to be poisons. They raise the bad LDL cholesterol levels and reduce beneficial HDL cholesterol levels (2).

The prostaglandin balance changes, and as a result inflammation occurs. There is increased evidence in diabetic patients that their cell membrane composition changes. Pro-inflammatory cytokines can cause pain in the dorsal root ganglions (3).

After reading all this information, it should be crystal clear that it is best to cut out all hydrogenated fat and margarines.

Conclusion

Never look back. Look forward to cutting out junk foods like refined sugar, empty starchy foods and processed foods. In addition when you cut out processed foods you have the benefit of eliminating hydrogenated fats, which contain free radicals and damage your arteries directly. When you remove the offending agents, the body will be able to repair itself.

Internet references

1. http://www.askdrray.com/prevent-cancer-cut-sugar/
2. https://www.ncbi.nlm.nih.gov/pubmed/?term=22135871
3. https://www.ncbi.nlm.nih.gov/labs/articles/21159431/

Is mouldy bread bad for me? Should I microwave it?

No, you do not know what mold type is growing on this slice of bread. For instance, aflatoxins are deadly (1).

Why take a risk? Throw the bread out. In future, keep bread in the fridge. It keeps longer.

Internet reference

1. https://en.wikipedia.org/wiki/Aflatoxin

Xylitol against tooth decay

Xylitol is a sugar replacement, which is also good for preventing cavities. I suggest you use either stevia, a plant sweetener or Xylitol with stevia to sweeten your coffee or tea rather than sugar. Xylitol gum is useful to prevent cavities of your teeth (1).

Internet reference

1. https://en.wikipedia.org/wiki/Xylitol

Consequences of a one-week fast

As long as you drink fluids, you would be fine, but you can expect to lose some pounds. If you do not drink fluids, you damage your kidneys, because your kidneys always need fluid or you would get dehydrated. People who go out into the desert with not enough to eat and drink face this dilemma. If people are lost and the rescue team finds them after 7 days, they will be doing well, as long as, they found a clean water source and drank. If they did not find water and did not have enough fluids along, the rescue team may find them dead. It is very simple: lack of fluid is more serious than lack of food.

Internet reference

1. https://www.mayoclinic.org/diseases-conditions/
dehydration/symptoms-causes/syc-20354086

Is there are difference between Irish butter and American butter?

The Irish butter won't have recombinant bovine growth hormone in it. This bovine growth hormone is used in dairy farming in the US to increase the milk production of dairy cows. At this point is still being investigated for possibly causing autoimmune diseases. Other countries have banned this hormone as illegal. It is not in Canadian and European dairy products. Since I'm not interested in being a guinea pig for a substance that is banned elsewhere, I will eat Irish butter, but not US butter. For the same reason I also refuse to buy American cheese.

Here is a reference that claims recombinant bovine growth hormone in milk would be harmless (1).

But the investigations are ongoing (2).

It appears that with the small amount of recombinant bovine growth hormone in US butter or milk it is possible that human growth hormone production could be suppressed, which is known to cause autoimmune diseases. Any such investigations are not being done, because it is inconvenient and costly. However, consumers are free to stick to Canadian milk products, Irish butter and European milk products. You also can switch to goat's milk, which is free from recombinant bovine growth hormone.

Internet references

1. https://www.cancer.org/cancer/cancer-causes/recombinant-bovine-growth-hormone.html

2. https://www.organicconsumers.org/sites/default/files/rbgh_harms_cows_fact_sheet.pdf

Chapter 17:

Digestion

Can you develop an ulcer in your stomach from not eating regularly?

1. Overview of how ulcers develop

Although people talk about "stomach ulcers", most peptic ulcers are actually duodenal ulcers, as they are located in the first part of the duodenum. When food leaves the stomach it is saturated with hydrochloric acid and it is forced around a C-shape curve of the duodenum.

The area at the beginning of this C-shape wall of the duodenum is the area that has the highest risk of developing a duodenal ulcer. Peptic ulcers can develop when the normal defense mechanisms of the mucosa lining are undermined.

This can be from the chronic use of anti-inflammatory medication for arthritis (NSAIDs). But it can also be from a bacterium called Helicobacter pylori, or for short: H. Pylori.

This bacterium has developed a remarkable ability to survive in the acidy milieu of the stomach and duodenum as it produces several enzymes, which enable it to neutralize the acid in its immediate micro surrounding.

It also produces mucolytic enzymes, which are capable of breaking down the superficial layer of the gastric and duodenal wall so that acid can now do the rest and erode the wall of the mucosa. A peptic ulcer (or simply ulcer) is a defect of the mucosal layer.

The term "peptic ulcer" comes from a time when physicians thought that ulcers would come from a combination of acid and the enzyme pepsin, which in combination would lead to the ulceration of the esophagus, stomach wall or duodenal wall. As pointed out above, we now know that defense mechanisms also play a tremendous role, as does a high secretion of ACTH and cortisol in the case of stress ulcers, which leads to a further weakening of these defense mechanisms. NSAIDs used for arthritis lead to a weakening of the repair mechanisms in the mucosal wall and increase the acidity on a cellular level, which means that the medication is "ulcerogenic" (it can cause ulcers).

Ulcers come in different forms. With NSAIDs it is often a multitude of erosions. These can be seen by a diagnostic procedure called gastroduodenoscopy. They are often located in the stomach, are very shallow and measure a few mm in diameter. Besides that there is a chronic duodenal ulcer, which may measure from 0.5 to 2 cm in diameter, and where the bacterium H. pylori may play a role as a chronic propagator. It is clear that any defect of the mucosa, which is full of blood vessels, can lead to bleeding ulcers.

2. Answering your question

It is true that if a patient with an ulcer does not eat regularly the acid in the stomach will corrode the stomach further when there is no food to digest in the stomach for a long time. Doctors usually recommend to the patient to take 5 small meals; this will bind the acid in the stomach by absorbing it in the food until it is digested and leaves the stomach. In the duodenum the milieu is alkaline and the acid is neutralized.

Next the doctor will recommend some medicine that will suppress acid formation and this will also help the body to heal. Triple antibiotics are often also recommended when it is proven that H. pylori is involved.

A well-researched remedy for stomach ulcers is licorice root. Licorice however contains glycyrrhetinic acid, which can elevate blood pressure. Scientists developed deglycyrrhizinated licorice tablets (DGL for short), which is very effective in relieving stomach ulcers, but has no side effect of elevating blood pressure. It comes in chewable tablets 380 to 400 mg of DGL per tablet. According to Murray (Ref. 1) the growth of H. pylori, the bacterium that causes difficult to heal ulcers, is inhibited by DGL. In head-to-head studies, which are cited by Ref. 1 DGL was more effective than Zantac, Tagamet or antacids. Two to three chewable DGL tablets taken between meals or 20 minutes before meals will heal ulcers within 8 to 16 weeks. The difference is that with DGL the ulcer is healed, while with standard medication described above it is only symptomatically suppressed, but will often flare up when the treatment is stopped. DGL stimulates the normal defense mechanisms of the stomach and duodenum, improves the protective substances that line the intestinal wall and improves blood supply to the intestinal lining. The result is that the lifespan of the intestinal cell is prolonged.

Book reference

Ref.1: Michael T. Murray, N.D.: "What the drug companies won't tell you and your doctor doesn't know" – The alternative treatments that may change your life – and the prescriptions that could harm you. Atria Books (subsidiary of Simon & Schuster Inc.), 2009 (page 73).

I am passing a lot of gas. What could be the cause?

Your bowel transit time may be too slow. You can test this by eating some corn. Swallow one or two bites of corn without chewing it well before. This becomes a marker. Note the time when you swallowed it and record the time when you notice it first in your stool. If this time lapse is more than 10 to 12 hours, you are constipated. Constipation is common. Other causes for gas can be foods. Some people react to beans or other legumes, which gave beans the nickname "the musical fruit". Food sensitivities can play a role as well. But constipation is even more common. Below you find a detailed description of constipation, borrowed from my NetHealthBook.com (1).

Constipation

Introduction

In general practice constipation is an important symptom that prompts patients to see their physician. There seems to be a lot of confusion in the general public about this topic. It starts by defining what a normal bowel movement is. There are enormous cultural differences. For instance, in Africa where the average population consumes a much larger amount of fiber in their food, the bowel movements are much bulkier.

Sir Dr. Burkitt, the famous English surgeon, examined bowel movements (stools) of African tribes in comparison to his English countrymen and came to the conclusion that in the Western world we need to remedy our constipation problem and cancer of the colon problem by eating more fiber.

He got it right: fiber is mainly treating the constipation (not preventing the cancer), but the chemicals that are also in the vegetables contain a multitude of natural anti-carcinogenic substances, which provide the powerful preventative action against colon cancer and many other cancers. Lycopene is one of these and is found in tomatoes and tomato products.

Sir Dr. Burkitt's observation that high bulk food (with vegetables and green leaves) prevents cancer is as valid today as it was in the early part of the 1900's. Next there is the question how often we should defecate. In a country where high fiber intake is the norm a daily or twice daily bowel movement is normal. However, in the Western world in highly developed countries the norm may be a bowel movement every other day. However, I do believe that this is unhealthy and is likely the reason for a high colon cancer rate. This is supported by the literature. To answer this difficult question of what a normal bowel movement rate would be, the answer is likely once every day, but those who eat a lot of vegetables may often get a second bowel movement during the day due to the extra bulk. Gastroenterologists now feel that twice per day is likely better than once.

Symptoms

There are different types of constipation.

1. Acute constipation

This is a condition where there is a sudden change from a normal bowel pattern to a bowel movement, which is 1 or 2 days delayed.

There might be bloatedness, a sense of fullness in the abdomen, particularly in the left lower abdomen and occasionally sharp stinging pains. This could be an ominous sign of a partial closing down of the colon lumen by a tumor. But it could be harmless in a patient that has become bedridden and there was less physical activity. It is also common when people travel. If this problem is persisting, a visit to the doctor is in order to rule out more serious problems like diverticulitis, head trauma, spinal cord lesion, or side effect of drugs (iron salts, pain pills, tranquilizers, sedatives).

2. Chronic constipation

Chronic constipation cases that start insidiously, but then remain despite taking a high fiber diet, make the doctor think about other underlying causes such as hypothyroidism (= low thyroid function) or other metabolic causes such as hypercalcemia and uremia from early kidney failure.

We find that elderly people become too inactive, which lowers the natural peristalsis of the gut, and this combined with poor eating habits and chewing problems because of dental problems is often responsible for the chronic constipation. Also the elderly often are on multiple drugs, all of which have a weak "anticholinergic" side effect, which translates into suppressing peristalsis chemically and resulting in constipation. Psychogenic factors and chronic depression as well as obsessive-compulsive behavior will often lead to a hyper awareness of one's own bowel pattern, which is unhealthy and needs to be addressed by counselling, once the doctor has ruled out any serious cause of the chronic constipation. The physician will examine with a rectal examination to rule out lower rectal lesions, hemorrhoids, anal fissures, benign polyps or cancer. The next test that gastroenterologists are using is a rectosigmoidoscopy and colonoscopy (= the Rolls Royce of colon exams). Occasionally a double Barium enema is done to look at the lining of the bowel wall.

If the problem is left alone, chronic constipation can lead to impaction, which sends the patient to the emergency room.

Treatment for constipation

Obviously the cause needs to be identified meaning that a physician needs to be consulted first. If no serious disease is found (cancer of the colon or rectum) and no metabolic disease is present that needs treatment, then the following steps likely will be recommended.

Treatment for constipation (simple steps that help)

• Food intake needs to be modified to include as much fresh and steamed vegetables as tolerated. This will lead to bulk in the colon and this will make the stool softer thus allowing it to pass through the rectum and anal canal easier. The other advantage of this simple step is that the bulkiness of the stool triggers the normal peristalsis the contents towards the rectum and out. By decreasing the passage time movement of the colon moving in the colon less water is absorbed, keeping the stool soft and pliable until it gets pushed through the anal canal. This is easily achieved by a diet which is rich in fruits and vegetables. Cereals containing bran, rolled oats (not instant) are also useful particularly for breakfast. Cut down on meat and fat consumption.

• A simple tool is an enema with lukewarm water (1500 ml or 50 oz.) in an enema bag without any additives in it. The person who gets the enema needs to lie on the left side so that the water can flow in easily. When inserting the nozzle into the anal canal, do not force it, but use a bit of Vaseline ointment to facilitate entry. The response usually comes within 5 to 10 minutes following the enema. It works by dilatation of the bowel wall, which leads to a reflex bowel contraction. This would be safe to take every day, but usually should not have to be taken more than two or three times per week even in chronic constipation. Some people may feel uncomfortable about this option, but the fact remains: it is the most effective method to get the bowels moving, and it gives immediate relief to the patient.

• Next, if this is not tolerated or does not appeal to the patient I would recommend a bulking agent such as psyllium (brand names: Prodiem Plain, Metamucil, Novo-Mucilax) and bran (Brand names: Kellogg's All Bran and Post's bran flakes). These are mild laxatives, which are safe to take every day and which will not make the patient hypokalemic.

• Osmotic agent: One or two tablespoons of sorbitol as a 70% solution is a hyperosmotic solution, which stays in the gut and draws water by osmosis into the colon. The bulking effect creates peristalsis and the water retention makes the stool softer. It takes often 1 or two days to get the full effect. There can be transient abdominal cramps until the stool is passed. One variation of this theme is to give sorbitol in a mix with other osmotic agents as a micro-enema in the form of Microlax (from Pharmacia and Upjohn).

• The "emergency break": Occasionally all of the above is simply too weak and the constipated person who normally is controlled with the above measures, simply could not go to the bathroom for several days. Bisacodyl (brand name: Dulcolax) and sennosides (brand names: Ex-lax Sugar Coated Pills and Senokot products) can be used on a one-time only basis. Increase your vegetable and fruit intake, cut down on refined foods, which are devoid of fiber.

I do not recommend any other products because they are expensive and not as effective. With mineral oil, for instance, there are dangers of aspiration with subsequent life threatening lipid pneumonia. Even with the suggestions above, one should always start on top and work with dietary changes first. It takes a few days to see the effect. Avoid the "emergency break" on a regular basis. This would be called laxative abuse and has devastating consequences as the body loses potassium and this in turn leads to secondary hyperaldosteronism (an increase of a mineralocorticoid hormone from the adrenal glands) and possible kidney damage (Bartter's syndrome).

The key to remember is that laxatives are only occasional emergency breaks that should not be taken daily.

Because of its role in nutrient absorption and body detoxification the digestive system plays a direct role in overall health and wellness. When the colon is unclean, waste and toxins can become trapped placing an extra strain on the detoxification organs and reducing immunity, thus causing illness.

Remember: "Do not abuse laxatives!"

The other fact is that when bisacodyl and sennosides are taken daily, they stop working after a few weeks because the body gets used to the medication. By treating these laxatives like an "emergency break only", the colon is responding to the medication when it is needed and all the other potential dangers like Bartter's syndrome and hypokalemia are not a problem.

Here is a site that shows an image of how bowel movements form in the colon (2).

Internet references

1. http://nethealthbook.com/digestive-system-and-gastrointestinal-disorders/constipation/
2. http://quickcare.org/gast/constipation.html

If I bring up yellow vomit, what does it mean?

1. It may simply mean you had too much fat in your last meal. In this case the bile, which normally flows downstream into the small bowel, can go upstream into the stomach to help digest your fatty meal. Once in the stomach, bile is very irritating, which causes vomiting.

2. There are more sinister diagnostic possibilities, if the condition persists and you no longer eat a fatty meal. The bile duct can get closed from a gallstone and vomiting bile could be a symptom of that. Alternatively a tumor in the head of the pancreas can block the common bile duct. It is advisable that you see a physician for proper diagnosis and treatment.

Chapter 18:

Doctor

As a doctor, have you diagnosed yourself and averted an emergency?

I was in my first year of medical school, listening to a lecture in physics (preclinical medical school subject), when I suddenly felt a sharp pain in my right lower abdomen. I also felt very nauseous. I suspected that I would have an early appendicitis (1).

Next I showed up at a clinic in the University Hospital of Tübingen University. The physician confirmed that I was suffering from acute appendicitis. Surgery had to be arranged right away. After seven days in hospital I could be discharged. They kept patients longer in hospital at that time than they do nowadays. It felt strange that I diagnosed my own condition before I ever had clinical lectures about it.

Internet reference

1. http://nethealthbook.com/abdominal-pain/right-lower-abdomen/appendicitis/

What stands out in your career as a doctor as a most memorable moment?

1. I had to look after a terminal brain cancer patient who was in his early 30's. The family wanted to treat him symptomatically at home. He had undergone chemotherapy and radiotherapy by the Cancer Clinic in the nearby city, but nothing helped and he was finally sent home to die. This was 5 months earlier. Desperate the family bought a large amount of Laetrile that was in fashion at the time. This is an apricot kernel extract that was often prescribed intravenously in Mexican cancer clinics (1).

2. I had read up on it, because patients wanted to try it in the terminal phases of cancer. I agreed that I would give it to this patient provided the family would sign a legal disclaimer document. It said that they understood that Laetrile was like a placebo medicine and could not be expected to cure his cancer.

3. The patient had been stable with his terminal brain cancer for the past 5 months. But lately he was drifting into longer and longer periods of unconsciousness. Christmas was fast approaching, and the relatives -some of them from far away- were gathering around this terminal cancer patient y. It was two days before Christmas when my patient slipped into a permanent coma. He was still breathing on his own, but I expected him to die any hour.

4. The family approached me whether I could give him a much higher dose of Laetrile than I had been given in the last few days. They still had a large supply and they were hoping that it would help at least for a few days so that the relatives could still enjoy the company of their loved one over the holidays. I had read in alternative medical literature that some physicians gave brain cancer patients up to 15 grams of Laetrile (this were 15 ampoules, given intravenously) daily. To my surprise, after receiving the

high dose of Laetrile, my patient came out of the coma. On the second day of the high dose of Laetrile he started talking and sitting up. I could not believe my eyes and ears, but it was happening right in front of me!

5. The family had a wonderful Christmas holiday. He stayed conscious until the New Year. But then he fell asleep and slipped back into a coma. He died in the first January days despite the continued Laetrile doses. He still had enjoyed the family and the family had enjoyed him.

6. I never had a satisfying medical explanation for this medical phenomenon. Was there brain edema, which for a period of time receded, lowering the pressure in his brain? Did the tumor shrink for a few days allowing him to wake up? It does not really matter. What counts is that the placebo worked very well, at least for a few days!

Internet reference

1. http://www.cancerresearchuk.org/about-cancer/cancer-in-general/treatment/complementary-alternative-therapies/individual-therapies/laetrile

Do you get compensated for a call: "Is there a doctor on the flight?"

I was once called: "Is there a doctor on the flight?" on an intercontinental flight between Frankfurt and Vancouver, BC.

I found that one other physician was also volunteering. The patient was an elderly woman who had fainted. She had not drunk enough water and was hypovolemic. She did not have any chest pain and no sign of a heart attack. She responded to intravenous fluids (a nurse had already started an IV with Ringer's lactate). Her blood pressure was fine. Between all of us we decided that she was fit to continue the flight.

Nobody compensated us, but the chief flight attendant thanked us very much. We were "Good Samaritans" who did the best we could under the circumstances. There is a legal advantage of not getting paid: if we had been wrong and the patient had died of a heart attack, we could have been sued for malpractice as we practiced medicine, had we been paid for the service. When the health professional does not get paid for the service, he/she cannot be sued because of some legal rules that have been established long time ago (the good "Samaritan clause").

Fortunately for all of us (the patient included) she was fine at the end of the flight.

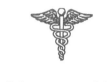

Chapter 19:

Exercise

How useful is cardiovascular exercise?

Regular cardio exercises prolong life by as much as 4.5 years, a study showed that is cited here (1).

The reason for this is that the heart will work more efficiently; the relatively small coronary arteries will open up more from the exercise. The end result is that there are less heart attacks or strokes. This adds to life expectancy. People who exercise regularly simply live longer and stay healthier.

To answer your question: regular cardio is NOT a waste of time; it makes you fit and adds to your life expectancy, as much as 4.5 years!

Internet reference

1. https://www.cancer.gov/news-events/press-releases/2012/PhysicalActivityLifeExpectancy

Does running or any other exercise help you to lose weight?

Exercising for weight loss will not yield spectacular results. You should exercise for heart and lung conditioning and for muscle conditioning. But to achieve weight loss the big emphasis should be put on dieting.

A study asked the question whether we can outrun dieting and the answer was "no". Weight loss can only be achieved to 8% from exercising, but to 92% by dieting (1).

I would suggest incorporating exercise into your weight loss program. It is needed for our cardio-vascular health and for our muscles. Just be aware that the higher contribution for weight loss will come from dieting, not from exercising.

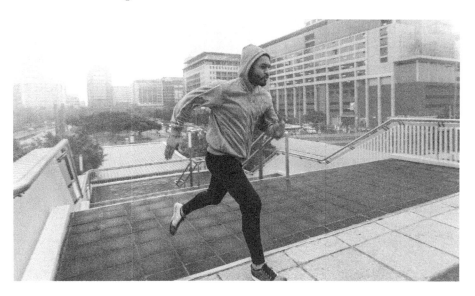

Internet reference

1. http://www.weightymatters.ca/2016/02/constrained-energy-expenditures-and-not.html

Could running marathons be dangerous for you?

Pheidippides, the first marathon runner died after he delivered a victory message (1).

Unfortunately many other marathon runners have experienced heart attacks or strokes, and many died also. 26.2 miles of high stress on your system due to continuous running takes all your reserves and can go beyond your limit to the point of damage.

Marathon runners, who do this often, say that they like the rush (endorphin high). But from a medical point of view there are negatives as well: the cartilage of the knees and hips gets overstressed, which often leads to osteoarthritis later in life. Many former marathon runners end up with hip and knee replacements. If the person has plaque in the coronary arteries, there may be spasms of the coronary arteries during the run, which can lead to a heart attack. When there is plaque in the brain vessels, the overexertion can lead to a stroke.

Regular physical exercise on a treadmill with a slope of 6% to 11% or going on an elliptical machine is preferable to hours of a strenuous marathon.

Internet reference

1. https://en.wikipedia.org/wiki/Pheidippides

Chapter 20:

Fate

What did you find sad about your mother and/or father?

1. You have to take life the way it comes. When I was a toddler, my mother had to talk to two French soldiers, as they wanted to occupy our house after WWII in Germany. When they saw me standing in a crib, they felt pity with us. My mother explained to them that my father was killed in WWII while working for the Red Cross (he was a physician) and she had to look after the family on her own. The soldiers took pity on her and occupied another house.

2. When I was 5 1/2 years old, my mother remarried an engineer. He was my stepdad and as I have never seen my own dad, I just accepted him as my father.

3. My mother came down with colon cancer and died at the age of 59. In those times (late 1970's) Germany did not use routine colonoscopies the way this is done now. Due to my family history I have had many colonoscopies and several colonic polyps were removed sparing me the headache of colon cancer.

4. My stepfather started to lose his memory in his mid 80's. He had to go into a home where Alzheimer's patients

were taken care of. He died at the age of 89. Even though this is a good age, it hurts to see your dad die. He supported me throughout my growing up years. Because of him I was able to go to medical school.

Conclusion

Life throws adversities at you. We need to be resilient and adapt to the changing world around us. There are other factors apart from family, such as the changing job environment etc. Whatever happens, we need to accept changes-the good and the not so good. Life is a picture with light and shadows.

Chapter 21:

Foot Problems

What is plantar fasciitis and how do you treat it?

Plantar fasciitis is one of the causes of heel pain (1). Deep inside the sole of the foot there is a flat sheet of connective tissue (called the "plantar fascia"), which helps to approximate the forefoot to the heel.

With prolonged standing the plantar fascia can get inflamed, and degenerative changes can take place close to the insertion of the plantar fascia near the heel bone, which is called plantar fasciitis. This leads to heel and foot pain and discomfort. This is usually associated with a heel cord contracture. At night the foot is usually plantar flexed (toe pointed downwards) and this aggravates the heel cord contracture. When the toes are bent upwards (dorsiflexed), the pain of plantar fasciitis is worsened. This is one of the diagnostic signs.

Flat foot and plantar fasciitis are unrelated. They are independent conditions.

Plantar fasciitis treatment consists of stretching exercises of the heel cord to improve postural factors. Any repetitive loading stress of the foot needs to be avoided such as running or prolonged standing. Plantar fasciitis shoes and plantar fasciitis night splints might help. Surgery for plantar fasciitis is an option only in less than 5% of cases and would consist of a plantar fascia release. Orthotics may be needed to redistribute some of the forces from the plantar fascia thus helping with the heel pain and foot heel pain associated with plantar fasciitis.

Internet reference

1. **http://www.wheelessonline.com/ortho/plantar_fasciitis**

Chapter 22:

Gut Disease

Is "gluten free" food healthy?

1. This is a big question. Since BASF (achemical company in Germany) has tinkered with the genetic makeup through chemical and radiation manipulation of wheat seeds in the 1960's and 1970's, the result called "Clearfield Wheat" has been marketed all around the world. This was done before the term GMO even became a discussion item. As a result modern wheat is 7-fold higher in gluten content than the old wheat varieties your grandparents consumed.

2. According to Ref. 1 among patients with irritable bowel syndrome (IBS) 4 to 5% have true gluten intolerance (celiac disease). In the general population (without IBS) the gluten sensitivity percentage is less than ¼ of that. On the other hand lactose intolerance in the US is found in 25% of all adults and in 35% to 45% of IBS patients. Another common food sensitivity is fructose and sorbitol intolerance, which occurs in about 40% of patients with IBS and about the same percentage in non-IBS controls. This means that if you leave out sorbitol and fructose, about 40% of people will find relief from abdominal cramps or

bloating. A common item that people chew on, according to Ref.1 is sorbitol-containing chewing gum. If this type of chewing gum is eliminated, 40% of people will feel better in their gut. Let us keep in mind that the majority of people with food sensitivities do not have gluten sensitivity, but lactose intolerance and allergies to fructose and sorbitol.

3. How do we know whether or not we are gluten sensitive? There are very sensitive blood tests that your doctor can order: Screening - Celiac Disease Foundation. Only 1% of people in the general population are gluten sensitive at this point. Just 30 years ago this number was 0.025%. 10 years ago 0.04% of people were thought to have gluten sensitivity. The difference may be due to improved sensitivity of the testing methods. But another factor is the new wheat, called Clearfield wheat mentioned above.

4. I think that the best prevention is to avoid wheat, as it is not the original any more. If you want to eat some grains, use brown rice, quinoa, buckwheat and organic corn that have not been genetically engineered. Instead of noodles use rice or quinoa noodles, shirataki or mung bean noodles (instead of rice noodles). Indulge in a variety of vegetables.

Conclusion

It is a good idea to avoid gluten as much as possible, even for people who are not allergic to it yet. Those who have a gluten allergy must avoid gluten at all costs as it will affect your gut barrier (leaky gut syndrome) and cause all kinds of autoimmune reactions including a skin rash (atopic dermatitis as part of celiac disease). Many gastroenterologists consider irritable bowel syndrome as the first indication towards gluten sensitivity. We need our bowel to absorb nutrients from our food, and we need that lifelong. We don't want chronic inflammation in our gut that interferes with absorption of nutrients. We cannot afford to take this too lightly!

Book reference

Ref.: 1. Rakel: Integrative Medicine, 3rd ed. Patrick J. Hanaway, MD: "Chapter40: Irritable Bowel Syndrome. Integrative Therapy". Copyright 2012 Saunders, An Imprint of Elsevier

Internet reference

1. https://celiac.org/celiac-disease/understanding-celiac-disease-2/what-is-celiac-disease/

Chapter 23:

Heart

Could we replace the heart with an artificial pump and live forever?

The artificial heart has been developed. But it is limited in terms of what it can do mechanically. It may work up to 2 years, but the person who depends on it still has to wait for a matching heart transplant. Even an artificial heart cannot replace the human heart on the long term, whether it is your own heart or a transplanted heart. The heart muscle is energized by a lot of mitochondria within each muscle fiber, and this is what allows the heart to function lifelong. But if you think that the heart pumping blood would be the solution to longevity, think again. You need flexible arteries that have hardly any arteriosclerotic changes in them, so nutrients and oxygen can reach every cell in the body to provide energy and nutrition. Your brain and the other vital organs (kidneys, liver, pancreas, digestive tract, hormone glands and more) need to function fully to enjoy a long life. It is unrealistic at this time to think that we can achieve immortality. This is just news talk. The highest we can expect to live, if we take good care of our bodies is thought at this time to be in the range of 110 to 120 years. This would be 30 to 40 years longer than most people live now. If you want to live a long, disease-free life, think prevention. Do not believe that a mechanical heart will give you a long and healthy life. Take care of your body now.

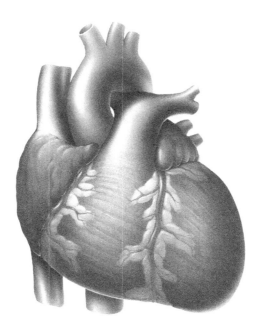

Chapter 24:

Heart Disease

What can I do to clean out my arteries and reduce my risk for heart disease?

Typically the person who has developed artery plaque is a person who ate too much sugar and starch and did not exercise regularly. They often also have some extra pounds of weight to carry around.
Sugar and starchy foods lead to oxidized LDL particles that are aggressively forming plaque. Sugar and starchy foods also increase triglycerides, a known risk factor for heart attacks and strokes.

1. My first recommendation therefore is to cut out sugar and to limit starchy foods (1).
2. Choose foods with a glycemic index of less than 55.
3. Exercise on a regular basis. This will bring your HDL cholesterol level up, which works on dissolving your own atherosclerotic plaques. HDL is the good cholesterol. It balances the LDL cholesterol, the bad cholesterol.
4. There are two vitamins that are important to consider: use 200 micrograms once daily of vitamin K2 and around 4000 to 5000 IU vitamin D3. Here I am explaining that calcium, vitamin D3 and vitamin K2 are needed for bone health (2).

5. It is good for your bones preventing osteoporosis, but also good for prevention of plaque formation in the arteries.

6. Forget technology. Cardiologists have procedures where they can clean out severe plaque from coronary arteries. But this tends to not hold up in time. The plaque reoccurs, when you do not change your lifestyle. In addition these surgical procedures are risky, occasionally even deadly.

Conclusion

As with many things in life, so it is with arterial plaque: it is back to basics! Pay attention to good nutrition and adopt a low glycemic diet. Also get into a regular exercise program of 30 minutes of a treadmill and 20 to 25 minutes of weight lifting using weight machines in a gym. If you have an exercise area in your home, it is even more convenient. Your heart does not take a break. Incorporate exercise into every day.

Internet references

1. http://www.whfoods.com/genpage.php?dbid=32&tname=faq
2. http://www.askdrray.com/calcium-vitamin-d3-and-vitamin-k2-needed-for-bone-health/

How do you assess the risk for heart disease in the elderly?

The pathophysiology of cardiovascular disease in the elderly is not any different than in the middle-aged person. The young person with no inborn abnormalities like homocysteinuria or obesity usually has no significant risk yet.

We talk about risk factors of cardiovascular disease:

1. High LDL cholesterol (the bad one) and low HDL cholesterol (the good one) are risk factors for heart attacks and strokes, as are high triglycerides.

2. High sugar consumption leads to the risks indicated under point 1. It is obvious that old or young alike should cut out sugar from the diet and severely reduce high glycemic foods in the diet. The reason is that sugar and starchy food oxidize LDL cholesterol, which subsequently becomes very aggressive and causes plugging up of coronary arteries and blood vessels to the brain and elsewhere in the body.

3. Oxidized LDL: As explained above sugar and starchy foods oxidize cholesterol. A Mediterranean diet including olive oil will stabilize your metabolism and protect LDL from being oxidized.

4. Elevated C-reactive protein: Dr. Paul Ridker published a landmark study in 2002 where he concluded that the blood test C-reactive protein was a reliable indicator to identify people who were at risk of developing a heart attack. It measures inflammation in the body. What is inflamed here is the lining of the arteries from oxidized LDL cholesterol. I hope you see a pattern. Some of these points are actually connected. Vitamin D3 and omga-3 fatty acids are counter balancing inflammation.

5. Excess insulin in people with diabetes, obesity or the metabolic syndrome: This leads to inflammation of the blood vessel wall and triggers accelerated hardening of the arteries. It also causes the brain arteries to get narrowed, and as a result the brain develops Alzheimer's and dementia. Alzheimer's is now called "type 3 diabetes". An overweight or obese person who cuts out sugar in the diet and exercises can often control excessive weight, lower insulin and normalize cognitive deficits.

6. Excess homocysteine: Some people are born with gene defects that program our cells to run abnormal biochemical

reactions in our metabolism. Correct methylation pathways are important for normal cell function (1).

However, if there is a methylation defect, abnormalities set in and homocysteine accumulates (2).

As we age, there is also a weakening of certain enzymes that are involved in the methylation pathway. With any of these enzyme defects you need to use appropriate supplements to normalize this metabolic defect. Vitamin B2, B6 and B12 supplementation will often stabilize methylation defects and homocysteine levels return to normal (3).

Methyl folate 1 mg per day is also very useful. Some people in older age cannot metabolize folate very well. This is important as severe, familial cardiovascular disease, where people often suffer heart attacks during the best years in their lives, can be postponed this way by several years or decades.

7. High blood pressure: Many people are not aware that high blood pressure is a disease where the linings of the arteries are inflamed and there is too little production of nitric oxide. Nitric oxide is a signalling substance contained in many vegetables, particularly in red beets. Nitric oxide is the body's tool to keep blood pressure normal by widening the diameter of arteries. High blood pressure leads to accelerated hardening of the arteries, because the oxidized LDL cholesterol gets deposited right under the diseased lining of the arteries. Just lowering the blood pressure with medications will not remove the other risk factors; they have to be addressed separately. The DASH diet has been developed to assist in lowering elevated blood pressure.

8. Vitamin D3 deficiency: Vitamin D3 is now considered to be a hormone, as all cells have receptors for this molecule. It has anti-inflammatory qualities. It helps in the prevention of heart attacks and strokes.

9. Low vitamin K2: Vitamin K2 and vitamin D3 co-operate in removing calcium from the blood and transporting it

into the bone. This way they both help in the prevention of osteoporosis. A co-factor in the prevention of osteoporosis is estrogen in women and testosterone in men.

10. Low free testosterone in men: Low free testosterone has been established as an independent risk factor for heart attacks and strokes. In the man there are a lot of testosterone receptors located in the heart and in the brain; this explains why with a lack of testosterone there is not only erectile dysfunction, but also the risk of developing a heart attack or a stroke.

11. Excess estrogen: When a women approaches menopause, her menstrual cycles can become irregular due to the fact that there are anovulatory cycles, and the progesterone production is starting to slow down. This hormonal state is called estrogen dominance, because estrogen dominates over progesterone. In other words, the ratio of progesterone over estrogen is less than 200 to 1 (progesterone/estrogen ratio) when saliva hormone levels are measured. This is a risk factor for hardening of the arteries. In males with a "beer belly" there is too much estrogen floating around due to an enzyme in fatty tissue, called aromatase. This enzyme manufactures estrogen out of testosterone and contributes along with other factors to causing heart attacks in overweight or obese men.

12. Stress and lack of sleep have been associated with increased rates of heart attacks and strokes.

13. Lack of regular exercise: this has been shown in many studies to be the cause of many diseases including cancer.

How can we protect ourselves from these risk factors?

As already indicated above, there are lifestyle issues that need to be addressed as follows.

1. First, adopt a healthy diet, such as the Mediterranean diet, which includes olive oil. No sugar, no bread, pasta, potatoes, and go extremely easy on certain fruit that is high in sugar, such as dried fruit, mango, bananas and grapes, because we do not want to oxidize our LDL cholesterol for reasons explained already.

2. Exercise regularly. If you like, go to a gym (my wife and I do this regularly). If you are insecure, ask a trainer initially to guide you through the exercise equipment. It really is not that difficult to do. You develop a routine that is good for you. Alternatively, you may want to go for a brisk walk, run or participate in dancing. If you get easily bored, rotate the activities, but do not skip days, let alone weeks! Remember that your heart works 24/7!

3. Take some vitamins and supplements: There are certain vitamins and supplements that will help prevent cardiovascular disease. The earlier we begin with this, the better: read my answer under "Vitamins and supplements" to this question: Are taking vitamins and supplements healthy or are they harmful?

Vitamin B2, B6, B12 and methyl folate were mentioned before. Take vitamin D3 in a good dose like 5000 IU per day or more and vitamin K2 (200 micrograms per day). Omega-3 supplements (EPA/DHA) are very useful to keep inflammation under control.

4. Have your hormones checked. Some doctors do not feel comfortable about this; maybe you want to see a naturopathic physician about it instead. Your body needs the hormone receptors satisfied by adequate bioidentical hormone levels; otherwise you age prematurely and give up body functions that you would rather keep. Normal hormone levels prevent osteoporosis, premature hardening of the arteries, Alzheimer's, erectile dysfunction and premature wrinkles.

Conclusion

All of these factors explained above are independent risk factors for developing hardening of the arteries, which affect mainly the heart, brain and kidneys. All you need is one of these factors, and you could develop a heart attack, stroke or kidney failure. You have no problem accepting a preventative maintenance program for your car. Think of having appropriate tests at least once a year done through your doctor. There are blood tests available to monitor hormone and vitamin levels, as well as the C-reactive protein and homocysteine levels. Take care of your heart and brain!

Internet references

1. http://www.dramyyasko.com/our-unique-approach/methylation-cycle/
2. http://www.foodforthebrain.org/alzheimers-prevention/methylation-and-homocysteine.aspx
3. https://www.dietitians.ca/Your-Health/Nutrition-A-Z/Vitamins/Functions-and-Food-Sources-of-Common-Vitamins.aspx

Are statins required by anybody with high cholesterol?

That's an interesting question: my answer is that there are hardly any health benefits from statins as outlined below, only for high risk cardiac patients.

How do statins work?

The statins are a group of drugs that inhibit an enzyme, called the hydroxymethylglutaryl–Coenzyme A (HMG-CoA), which leads to a lowering of cholesterol, specifically a fraction known as the LDL cholesterol. The success story of lovastatin (Mevacor) led to a flurry of new HMG-CoA reductase inhibitors (cholesterol lowering drugs) such as fluvastatin (Lescol), pravastatin (Pravachol), simvastatin (Zocor), atorvastatin (Lipitor), and rosuvastatin (Crestor) in the late 1980's and the 1990's. Collectively it is now a 26 billion industry in annual sales (1).

Later investigations showed that there were other mechanisms by which statins helped, namely they were found to decrease the inflammatory reaction, which can be measured by lowering of the C-reactive protein. However, there are significant side effects in about 1 to 3% of people who take this medication, particularly an inflammation of liver cells (evident from elevation of liver enzymes) and a myopathy, which is a painful muscle condition (Ref. 1). This latter fact, which can occur in as many as 33% of the population at large (particularly the exercise minded) has limited the use of statins in competitive athletes where myopathies can occur in as many as 75% of athletes treated with statins (Ref.2). The reason for that is that the muscles of athletes cannot keep up with the demands put on them when they are kept in check by the HMG-CoA reductase inhibitors. On the other hand statins have prevented heart attacks and strokes. Also deaths from heart attacks and strokes have been prevented in 25 % of patients who were put on statins (Ref.1). Nevertheless, simple supplements that have no side effects can do the same or do even better (see below).

The lack of cholesterol synthesis by the body's cells when statins are given, leads to an expression of more LDL receptors on the cell surfaces. LDL binds to these receptors and enters the cells, which removes the circulating high risk LDL fraction of cholesterol from the blood thus causing a drop in LDL cholesterol. All of the side effects of statins can be explained as a result of the slow-down of organ functions (brain, muscles, gut, adrenal glands, etc.) as cholesterol synthesis is reduced (2).

New information about cholesterol

Another important piece of research (April 2013) comes from Spain where doctors followed a group of 7447 patients with a high cardiovascular risk who were put on a Mediterranean diet with olive oil, a Mediterranean diet with nuts or a regular diet (3).

The end point was death from heart attack or stroke. After 4.8 years the study had to be interrupted as the Mediterranean groups showed a significant survival advantage over the group on a regular diet.

Ref. 4 cited literature evidence that statins cause a 48% increased risk to develop diabetes in postmenopausal women who take statins. It also cites compelling evidence that diabetes patients are twice as likely to develop Alzheimer's disease within 15 years and are 1.75 times more likely to develop any kind of dementia in the same time period.

Dr. Seneff from the Computer Science and Artificial Intelligence Laboratory at MIT explains in great detail that statins effectively reduce cholesterol synthesis in the liver, which in turn starves the brain of one of its main nutrients explaining why patient develop Alzheimer's disease and dementia as a result of statin treatment (4).

The lessons to be learnt from these clinical trials are that you want to offer your brain enough cholesterol and healthy fat to have a normal metabolism. Fortunately, what's good for your heart is also good for your brain. Conversely avoid statins, if you can and try alternatives first. Ref. 4 explains that for years the experts had the wrong theory that low fat/high carb was what would be good for your heart and brain, but the opposite is true: what is good for your heart and brain is a high healthy fats/low refined carb diet.

Make sure to have blood tests that pay more attention to your fasting insulin level and cholesterol levels. Your fasting insulin should be low (no insulin resistance); the ratio of total cholesterol to HDL cholesterol should be less than 3.4 (low risk for heart attacks or strokes) and that the hemoglobin A1C level should be low (4.8 to 5.6%, ideally less than 4.5%), which means you are not diabetic.

How alternative treatment can save you from heart attacks

Lifestyle treatment through dietary intervention, moderate exercise, and weight loss has been somewhat neglected by mainstream medicine, but is now recognized in regular textbooks of medicine as first-line treatment (Ref. 3). Most patients can lower LDL cholesterol by 10 to 15% through a change in diet. High-risk patients with established heart disease (narrowing of coronary arteries) require a drop of 30 to 60% of LDL cholesterol; this high-risk patient group may need an addition of a statin. In patients with metabolic syndrome or diabetes high triglycerides are often present and will respond to decreased intake of simple sugars, alcohol, and calories (Ref.3). Total calorie intake should be adjusted according weight. The goal is reaching the normal body mass index range (BMI of 20 to 25), after which it is important to maintain the weight. The total fat intake should be around 25%-35% of the total calorie intake. Specifically, saturated fat needs to be less than 7% of total calories, polyunsaturated fat up to 10% of total calories and monounsaturated fat up to 20% of total calories. Healthy fats according to Ref. 4 are extra-virgin olive oil, organic butter, avocados, olives, nuts, nut butters and cheese (except for blue cheeses). Other healthy fats are sesame oil, coconut oil, and the oils found in seeds like flaxseed, sunflower seeds, pumpkin seeds and chia seeds. Note that trans-fats (such as in margarine and baked goods) are a "no-no" as it leads to free radicals in your body, which would accelerate the hardening of your arteries. Complex carbohydrates from vegetables and fruit are the main source of total calories providing 50%-60% of the total calories. Fiber intake needs to be 20-30 grams per day. Protein intake should be about 15% of total calories. Fat should provide 25% to 35% of the total calories per day. Cholesterol intake should be less than 200 mg per day. You may want to consider the use of plant sterols (2 grams per day) to enhance LDL cholesterol lowering. Physical activity from moderate exercise should expend at least 200 kcal per day (better 300 kcal).

Which supplements prevent heart attacks and strokes?

There are several nutrients that have been shown to be powerful preventers of heart attacks and strokes. I will review them briefly here (based on Ref. 2):

1. Coenzyme Q10 (CoQ10): The cells lining the arteries are only working well when their mitochondria are working properly producing chemical energy in form of ATP. CoQ10 is an important component of the mitochondrial metabolism; it is also the only fat soluble antioxidant that gets absorbed into the LDL particles where it protects these from oxidation. Statins suppress CoQ10 synthesis, and as a result patients on statins need to take CoQ10 supplements daily to counteract this. However, anybody who is healthy now should take CoQ10 as a daily supplement for prevention. I take 400 mg per day.

2. Vitamin E (tocopherols): this fat soluble vitamin is an antioxidant and has been praised in the past as being heart supportive, was subsequently bad-mouthed by some conservative physicians, but lately has been validated

as important for heart health. It turns out that there are 8 different types of tocopherols, with the alpha tocopherol being the most known, but gamma tocopherol is the one you want to make sure you are also getting with your balanced vitamin E supplement every day, as this is the one that is a powerful anti-inflammatory. Simply ask staff at your health food store for a vitamin E supplement with gamma tocopherol. Take 400 IU per day (of the mix).

3. Curcumin: This is a powerful heart and brain protector combining three different mechanisms in one; it is reducing oxidative stress, is an anti-inflammatory and counters the process that threatens to destroy the lining of the arteries. One study on healthy volunteers showed a reduction of 33% in lipid oxidation, a 12% reduction of total cholesterol and an increase of 29% of the protective HDL cholesterol when 500 mg of curcumin was taken only for 7 days (Ref.2). This is the daily dose I would recommend for prevention of heart attacks and strokes.

4. Polyphenols: Flavonoids are the largest group among the polyphenols contained in such common foods as vegetables, fruits, tea, coffee, chocolate and wine. Over 130 studies have been done on humans showing improvement of the lining of the arteries (endothelial functioning) and lowering of blood pressure. Polyphenol consumption has been associated with a lower risk of mortality from heart attacks. Eat a Mediterranean type diet or a DASH diet and you will automatically get enough polyphenols with your food. However, resveratrol, the powerful red wine polyphenol, warrants a separate daily supplementation as it prevents LDL oxidation in humans (Ref.2). Take about 250 mg of it daily.

5. Niacin/nicotinic acid: This supplement comes as "flush-free niacin" and also as extended release niacin; it can raise the beneficial HDL cholesterol by 30 to 35%

when higher doses of 2.25 grams per day are used. In a metaanalysis of 7 studies it has been shown to significantly reduce heart attacks and transient ischemic attacks (precursor syndrome before developing a stroke). Niacin can change the small particle LDL into a large particle size LDL, which is less dangerous. Niacin has also been shown to reduce oxidation of LDL, which stops the atherosclerotic process. For a healthy person 500 mg per day of flush-free niacin is adequate.

6. Fish oil (omega-3-fatty acids): Because heart attacks are due to an inflammatory process and high LDL cholesterol is thought to be only a secondary phenomenon, it is very important to have this additional tool of an important anti-inflammatory supplement. In the past it was still safe to eat fish fairly frequently per week. But with mercury and carcinogenic PBC's all congregating in the ocean waters, it is no longer safe to consume fish in large quantities. The remedy to this situation is molecularly distilled (or pharmaceutically pure) EPA/DHA supplements. EPA stands for eicosapentaenoic acid or omega-3 fatty acid. DHA is the acronym for docosahexaenoic acid. Fish oil supplements at a dosage of 3.35 grams per day of EPA plus DHA were shown to reduce triglycerides by up to 40%, equally to Lipitor or even more effective, but without the statin side effects. The amount of the dangerous small dense LDL is also being reduced with fish oil. Fish oil supplements have reduced the mortality from heart attacks and strokes and led to a higher survival from non-fatal heart attacks. At the same time these preventative fish oil doses will also treat and prevent arthritis.

7. Other useful supplements: Soluble fiber from psyllium, pectin, beta-glucans and others have been shown in clinical trials to reduce LDL cholesterol by binding bile salts in the gut (interrupting the enterohepatic pathway). Plant sterols

(usually sold as sterol esters) are recognized by the FDA as reducing the risk of coronary heart disease, if taken in high enough amounts (2.4 grams of sterol esters per day). There are other useful supplements like artichoke extract, pomegranate, soy protein, Indian gooseberry (Amla), garlic and pantethine (vitamin B5) that have been proven to be of benefit in terms of prevention of heart attacks and strokes. It would be too lengthy to get into more details here.

Conclusion

Statins are important for end stage cardiac patients. However, as mentioned, they also have significant side effects. Lifestyle factors are more powerful on the long term in terms of preventing heart attacks and strokes.

Exercise creates more nitric oxide production by the lining of the arteries, which opens up arteries and prevents spasms. A proper diet with as many of the proven vitamins and other support factors will control inflammation and oxidation of LDL cholesterol particles as explained. This will prevent heart attacks and strokes, as has been shown in many clinical trials. Only patients who come from families with genetically high cholesterol or high triglycerides and those patients who had heart attacks and strokes should be exposed to statins, as they are at a higher risk of developing a heart attack or stroke. They need all of the help they can get in addition to the lifestyle factors. Most other patients and the public at large will do quite well without statins (no side effects of diabetes, Alzheimer's and muscle pains). People with high borderline cholesterol levels have better cognitive function as this study showed (5). And, yes, a diet high in healthy fats, but low in refined carbs is what your brain and heart need (the opposite of what you have thought, see Ref. 4).

Book references

1. Bonow: Braunwald's Heart Disease – A Textbook of Cardiovascular Medicine, 9th ed. © 2011 Saunders.

2. Life Extension: Disease Prevention and Treatment, Fifth edition. 130 Evidence-Based Protocols to Combat the Diseases of Aging. © 2013

3. Melmed: Williams Textbook of Endocrinology, 12th ed. © 2011 Saunders.

4. David Perlmutter, MD: "Grain Brain. The Surprising Truth About Wheat, Carbs, And Sugar-Your Brain's Silent Killers." Little, Brown and Company, New York, 2013.

Internet references

1. http://haydeninstitute.com/medication-side-effects/pfizer-ads-come-clean-about-lipitor
2. http://www.webmd.com/cholesterol-management/side-effects-of-statin-drugs#1 (pull down to side effects in this link).
3. http://www.nejm.org/doi/full/10.1056/NEJMoa1200303
4. http://people.csail.mit.edu/seneff/alzheimers_statins.html
5. http://journals.lww.com/psychosomaticmedicine/Abstract/2005/01000/Serum_Cholesterol_and_Cognitive_Performance_in_the.4.aspx

Chapter 25:

High Blood Pressure

Are there treatments other than drugs to treat high blood pressure?

Most cases of high blood pressure (hypertension) are simply there without a particular cause. It used to be called "essential hypertension", a fancy name meaning, "essentially, we do not know the cause". The doctor will start treatment with drugs to bring high blood pressure down (1). Before that the doctor is supposed to ask you to make a good effort to change your life style (cutting out additional salt, exercising, weight loss), but this is often glossed over and drugs are used right away. Drugs for hypertension are not harmless; here are some of the side effects (2).

The medical textbooks are not very clear on what causes high blood pressure. With renal causes (narrowing of a renal artery) a stent can be placed, the cause is treated and the blood pressure normalizes. As indicated, essential hypertension is the name for the majority of other cases of high blood pressure where officially no cause is known. Patients are usually put on life-long blood pressure-lowering medications, often several drugs in combination, to bring the blood pressure down to 120 over 80.

Despite the notion that we do no know the cause of high blood pressure, we do know that a number of factors can contribute to developing high blood pressure: too much salt in the diet, too much nicotine from smoking and too much alcohol consumption (3).

A lack of nitrates from green vegetables can cause high blood pressure as well. Nitrates are necessary for the body to produce nitric oxide, a powerful messenger that dilates blood vessels lowering blood pressure (4).

It is produced every second by the lining inside the walls of your arteries. Greens and vegetables, particularly beets, provide nitrates for nitric oxide production (5).

Nitric oxide, along with omega-3-fatty acid and prostaglandins are important in relaxing the arterial walls, thus lowering high blood pressure.

We also know that in diabetes and obesity high blood pressure is very common, because inflammatory substances circulate in the blood, which interfere with the normal production of the blood pressure lowering nitric oxide.

Treating high blood pressure with the conventional drugs will mask the real underlying causes.

The DASH diet has helped a lot of people to get their blood pressure under control (6).

However, the limiting point in that diet is the amount of grains that are allowed. In my opinion, wheat and grains, starches and sugar are all empty calories and only stimulate your appetite because of the high leptin and gliadin content from wheat and wheat products. According to the cardiologist, Dr. William Davis, cutting these out will cure not only many cases of hypertension, but also diabetes and obesity. Many physicians have criticized him, but in my opinion his work is on solid researched ground.

If a patient honestly gives lifestyle changes a try, many side effects and deaths from antihypertensive drugs could be avoided. It is also important that the patient carefully monitors his daily blood pressure if despite all effort the readings are not reaching a normal level, it is time to use a blood pressure lowering medication (7).

Internet references

1. http://www.mayoclinic.org/diseases-conditions/high-blood-pressure/basics/definition/con-20019580
2. http://www.webmd.com/hypertension-high-blood-pressure/guide/side-effects-high-blood-pressure-medications#1
3. http://www.mayoclinic.org/diseases-conditions/high-blood-pressure/expert-answers/blood-pressure/faq-20058254
4. https://en.wikipedia.org/wiki/Nitric_oxide
5. http://www.qmul.ac.uk/media/news/items/smd/95990.html
6. http://www.mayoclinic.com/health/dash-diet/HI00047
7. https://www.ncbi.nlm.nih.gov/pubmed/11141143

Is the wall of the left heart chamber always thicker than the right one?

The body is designed to have a low-pressure system for the right heart, the pulmonary arteries and veins; and a high-pressure system for the left heart chamber and the body circulation.

There is a condition where the right ventricle is thicker than normal, in the case of pulmonary high blood pressure.

The medically more correct name for pulmonary high blood pressure is "arterial pulmonary hypertension" or simply "pulmonary hypertension". Indiscriminate prescribing patterns of Fen-Phen, a medication that was used as diet pills and consisted of two weight loss medications in combination, led to another form of hypertension, pulmonary hypertension, as a serious side effect.

It was a rare complication, but so significant that the FDA decided to withdraw the products from the market. Fenfluramine and phentermine in concert were more effective in weight loss than each alone, but the side effects added up alarmingly.

They led in some cases to fibrotic permanent changes of heart valves and the lining of the pulmonary vessels. This led to breathing problems, high blood pressure inside the pulmonary vessels and to congestive heart failure resistant to the normal medical therapy resulting in premature death.

More info about high blood pressure here (1).

Internet reference

1. http://nethealthbook.com/cardiovascular-disease/high-blood-pressure-hypertension/pulmonary-high-blood-pressure/

Chapter 26:

Hormones

Is estrogen present in the male body?

Below I will tell you what the Massachusetts General Hospital study found regarding estrogen in men. To give you a preview: a small amount of estrogen is necessary for sexual desire in a male and will also prevent obesity (more below).

Introduction

Much has been written about what happens when women get into menopause. This begs the question: do men experience a change of life? As a matter of fact, they do. It is called "andropause", and they can experience problems as a result. Here is a study from the Massachusetts General Hospital in Boston, MA, which was published in the New England Journal of Medicine (Sept. 2013) describing in detail what happens when men get into andropause, which is the male equivalent of the menopause (1).

We know from other studies that in obese men testosterone is converted into estrogen because of the enzyme aromatase that converts testosterone into estrogen resulting in erectile dysfunction and loss of sex drive. In lean men above the age of 55 there is a true testosterone reduction because the testicles produce less testosterone. This results in less sex drive, moodiness and lack of energy. But these men will do well with bioidentical testosterone replacement.

Main findings of the Massachusetts General Hospital study

1. Testosterone was responsible for thigh muscle development and leg press strength, for erectile function and sexual desire.

2. Surprisingly, estradiol (the main estrogen component in both sexes) plays a significant part in sexual desire in the male. This became particularly apparent in the post-andropause male who desired hormone replacement. When bioidentical testosterone is used to replace what's missing there was no problem with sexual desire or erectile function as a small amount of the testosterone was aromatized into estradiol. The researchers were able to measure both testosterone and estradiol levels.

3. Here is a surprising fact: a lack of estrogen leads to abdominal obesity. This could also be verified by hormone measurements.

4. In the past doctors used synthetic testosterone products like methyltestosterone, danazol, oxandrolone, testosterone propionate, testosterone cypionate or testosterone enanthate. The problem with these synthetic testosterone products is that the body cannot metabolize a portion of them into estrogen that is desirable for a normal sex drive, so the testosterone compounds alone are not doing their job as well as the bioidentical testosterone that the body can aromatize.

In obese men the problem is that there is too much estrogen in the system, which leads to a disbalance of the hormones in the male with a relative lack of testosterone. Overweight and obese men produce significant amounts of estrogen through aromatase located in the fatty tissue. Aromatase converts testosterone and other male type hormones, called androgens, into estrogen. Excessive levels of estrogen cause breast growth, muscle weakness, lead to abdominal fat accumulation, heart disease and strokes. Dr. Lee described years ago what happens in men who enter andropause as indicated under this link (2).

Testosterone to estrogen ratio

Dr. Lee indicated that in his opinion saliva hormone testing is more reliable than blood tests (Ref. 1). One of the advantages of doing saliva hormone tests of estrogen and testosterone is that you can calculate directly the ratios of these two hormones. In hormonally normal younger males the testosterone to estrogen ratio is larger than 20 – 40 (Ref.2). The testosterone to estrogen ratio in obese men is typically less than 20 meaning it is too low. But lean men in andropause produce too little testosterone, and their testosterone to estrogen ratio is also less than 20, because they may still have enough estrogen in their system from aromatase in the fatty tissue, but they are lacking testosterone due to a lack of its production in the testicles (Ref. 1 and 2).

When a man in andropause is given bioidentical hormone replacement with a testosterone gel or bioidentical testosterone cream, this is absorbed into the blood and body tissues and then partially metabolized into a small amount of estrogen. This can be seen when saliva hormone tests are done; a higher level of testosterone is detected and much lower estrogen level so that the testosterone to estrogen ratio is now 20 to 40 or higher and the affected person will no longer be the "grumpy old man" that had been a source of distress to his partner before.

This New England Journal of Medicine study is important because it confirmed what anti-aging physicians had been saying for years: a small amount of estrogen is necessary for the male for bone health as estrogen receptors will regulate the bone density, it also helps for a normal sex drive. The same is true for women: a small amount of the opposite hormone (testosterone) will help a woman's sex drive, but she needs the right mix of progesterone to estrogen (a progesterone to estrogen ratio of 200:1 using saliva tests) to feel perfectly normal as a woman.

Health and well being of a man depend on normal testosterone levels

It is important to realize that testosterone is not only supporting a man's sex drive and libido. Key organs like the heart, the brain and blood vessels contain testosterone receptors as well. The body of a man was designed to respond to testosterone all along. It is when testosterone production is no longer keeping up that premature aging becomes apparent, as the target organs do no longer receive the proper signals (3).

A healthy heart in a man depends on regular exercise and testosterone stimulation whether he is young, middle aged or old. The same is true for the lining of the arteries where testosterone receptors are present to help with the normal adjustment to exercise and relaxation. The brain cells have receptors for all of the sex hormones, and in a man they are used to higher levels of testosterone and lower levels of progesterone and estrogen. If you take the balance away, the aging man will feel miserable and grumpy. Depression will set in. Here is a brief review how one man's life has been changed by testosterone replacement (4).

It becomes clear that bioidentical hormone replacement is not just a matter of replacing one hormone, you need to pay attention to all of the hormones. Lifestyle issues enter the equation as well.

Internet reference

http://www.dcnutrition.com/miscellaneous-nutrients/male-hormones/

Is testosterone effective?

1. If bio identical testosterone used to only replace what is missing, then testosterone replacement works. All the major organ systems in a male have testosterone receptors. For optimal function these receptors need to be stimulated at all times. But in older men over the age of 55 or 60 blood tests show missing testosterone. A total testosterone level under 500 ng/dL means that the man needs testosterone replacement. Any doctor can either prescribe topical testosterone cream or injectable testosterone to bring back the testosterone level to normal. This will protect the heart from heart attacks, protect from strokes, give the man stamina and restore his sex drive to normal.

2. If you wonder whether testosterone compounds like androgen steroids work for bodybuilding, I have to disappoint you. There will be muscle bulk increase in certain areas of the body: But you run the risk of getting a heart attack, a stroke or liver cancer with these synthetic testosterone products. The problems is that your testosterone receptors cannot read the synthetic testosterone-like compounds and some of the natural testosterone action is blocked in key organs like the liver, the kidneys, the heart and brain.

Conclusion

In an aging male, bioidentical hormone replacement with testosterone is a God-sent. It has the potential of allowing him to live for 10–15 years longer and stay well. For this reason it can be considered an anti-aging agent. But synthetic testosterone compounds for bodybuilding should be outlawed. As explained, they are dangerous compounds. They shorten the lives of their users. They often end up with heart attacks at a young age and can also die from liver cancer.

Book references

Ref. 1: John R. Lee, MD: "Hormone Balance for men- what your doctor may not tell you about prostate health and natural hormone supplementation". 2003 by Hormones Etc.

Ref. 2: George Gillson, MD, PhD, Tracy Marsden, BSc Pharm: "You've Hit Menopause. Now What?" 2004 Rocky Mountain Analytical Corp. Chapter 9: Male Hormone Balance (p.118-148).

Ref. 3: Dr.Schilling's book, March 2014, Amazon.com: "A Survivor's Guide To Successful Aging":
https://www.amazon.com/Survivors-Guide-Successful-Aging-Christina/dp/1494765330/ref=sr_1_1?ie=UTF8&qid=1398270215&sr=8-1&keywords=books+dr.+schilling

Internet references

1. http://www.nejm.org/doi/full/10.1056/NEJMoa1206168?query=featured_home&#t=articleDiscussion

2. https://www.johnleemd.com/testosterone-booster-male-menopause.html
3. http://agelessandwellness.com/services-for-men/guide-to-mens-hormone-health/
4. http://www.wpbf.com/article/hrt-not-just-a-women-s-health-issue/1321937#!IIBrG

Why does testosterone production in a male decrease with age?

All hormone glands show aging including the testicles of a man. It starts with the pineal gland where melatonin production is clearly reduced from age 20 onwards.

Similarly, with human growth hormone production there is a clear reduction of production by the anterior pituitary gland at the age of 30 and beyond. With regard to testosterone production there is a critical limit reached by the age of 65 to 74.

This is when the total blood testosterone level reaches 500 ng/dL or less. 500 ng/dL is the limit under which testosterone replacement needs to be considered. Otherwise a male will age prematurely, have a higher risk of heart attacks and strokes and have a higher probability of developing prostate cancer.

Conclusion

I have only discussed three examples of declining hormone production due to aging. Anti-aging physicians monitor all hormones by blood and/or saliva hormone tests. If hormones are lower than acceptable, they are replaced up to physiological levels with bioidentical hormones. This rejuvenates the body. A person can live 10 to 15 years longer with bioidentical hormone replacements compared to controls that do not get hormones replaced. This is not only about living a few years longer; it is just as important that these years are years of wellness.

How can I increase testosterone and lower estrogen in my blood?

1. You may expect me to say that exercise would increase testosterone. But this is a marginal effect and not reliable. You may also expect me to recommend a certain diet to influence testosterone or estrogen levels. Again, this is disappointing because every person reacts differently.

2. The only thing that is reliable is to measure blood levels as a baseline test. If in a male the total testosterone level is greater than 500 ng/dL, no replacement is necessary, because the body makes enough testosterone. If it is less than 500 ng/dL, replacement is necessary.

3. In a male it is important to have a total testosterone to estrogen ratio of 20 or more. If this is not the case (meaning that estradiol is too high), indole-3-carbinole is useful to take. This is the effective agent in broccoli and other cruciferous vegetables that metabolizes estrogen and lowers the risk for breast cancer in women and prostate cancer in men. If men have too much estrogen they suffer from erectile dysfunction. This happens in obese men as the enzyme aromatase that is produced in fatty tissue turns male hormones into estrogen. Too much estrogen in males also causes heart attacks and strokes. Exercise, weight loss and indole-3-carbinole can reverse and normalize this.

4. In women things are a bit more complicated. There is another hormone, namely progesterone, which in relation to estrogen should have a ratio of 400:1 or more. Women need a little bit of testosterone to enjoy intimacy. But they need to watch that they do not overproduce estrogens. If their

estrogen levels are too high, they are at risk of developing heart attacks and strokes. They are more likely to suffer from migraines. They have a risk of forming cysts in their breasts and breast cancer. They also are more likely to get heavy periods and develop fibroids. In addition uterine cancer is a danger after several years of high estrogen levels. See your doctor to get checked out.

More info can be found here (1).

Internet reference

1. http://www.askdrray.com/testosterone/

I was diagnosed with hypothyroidism and started on levothyroxine. How long before I will be better?

You need to talk to your doctor. Levothyroxine is T3, but the body produces a mix of T3 and T4. I had patients who were put on Synthroid (which is T4) and others who were put on Levothyroxine (T3) and they both did not get fully controlled with their symptoms. I put these people on Armour, which is a T3/T4 mix, and they normalized within 1 month.

There are many physicians who still will insist on replacing with "pure" thyroid hormones, either T3 or T4. I learnt at many A4M conferences in Las Vegas (I go to their yearly anti-aging conferences regularly) that you must give the body what it produces itself, which is a mix of T3 and T4. Next your physician will criticise that Armour is porcine thyroid extract, which would not be standardized. You can tell him or her that this is bogus. The FDA has done analyses. Each 30 mg tablet of Armour contains 30 mg of standardized thyroid extract. And each 60 mg tablet of Armour contains 60 mg. Armour thyroid is a standardized extract.

With Armour treatment your TSH level should come down to between 0.2 and 2.0. This is the target range and is another bone of contention. Conventional medicine says a TSH below 5.0 would be adequate. This point was discussed at many A4M conferences. The Life Extension Magazine has discussed this point as well. You must bring TSH down much below 5.0, because high TSH is a carcinogenic (cancer producing). I repeat again what various professors at various A4M conferences have said: "With treatment of hypothyroidism the TSH level should come down to between 0.2 and 2.0". This is the target level (1).

Internet reference

1. **https://academic.oup.com/jcem/article/98/9/3584/2833082**

Does flaxseed consumption decrease testosterone levels?

Lignans contained in flaxseed are like a weak estrogen compound. This is not good for males in too high a dose. Here is a blog from a dodge ball player who ate 10 tablespoons of ground flaxseed per day and halved his testosterone level doing this. "Testosterone and Flax: A Male Nightmare? (1)"

Another website reviewed the effect of flaxseed on women as there is a concern whether it would cause breast cancer. But in animal experiments and human observations this fear is not justified, as 2 to 3 tablespoons of ground flaxseed actually reduced the risk for breast cancer (2).

As this link explains flaxseed acts like a selective estrogen receptor modulator, or SERM, similar to Tamoxifen.

Many people want to take ground flaxseed as a source of omega-3 fatty acids. Molecularly distilled marine omega

3 capsules are probably the safest source of omega-3 fatty acids or molecularly distilled Krill oil.

To answer your question: in males consumption of flaxseed will likely reduce testosterone in higher doses. More than 2 tablespoons per day should not be consumed by males. In women there seems to be no concern and it may actually prevent breast cancer.

Internet references

1. https://www.nuhs.edu/christian/2011/3/1/testosterone-and-flax-a-male-nightmare/
2. https://www.oncologynutrition.org/erfc/hot-topics/flaxseeds-and-breast-cancer/

What is unexpected when you get old?

Hormone deficiencies are what many people do not expect.

1. You get muscle aches and pains and your energy is missing. Your sleep is getting shallower and you wake up during the night several times. Your doctor suspects that you may have a hormonal problem. Your thyroid-stimulating hormone (TSH) is 14.6 and your T3 and T4 hormones are low. After some thyroid hormones (Armour, which is a mix of T3 and T4) your energy comes back, your muscle aches and pains disappear and you sleep again the way you used to do it.

2. A man who likes to have his regular sex life may feel frustrated. He is approaching his end sixties, and there is a problem in this department. Erections are not what they used to be, and he finds it more difficult to reach orgasm. Instead of every 2 days, he only wants sex every 3 to 4 days-or even less. He sees his family doctor who sends him for lab work and orders a testosterone level. A low level

of testosterone shows up on a blood test. The doctor starts him on twice weekly testosterone self-injections. Within 2 weeks his regular sex life returns, quite to the astonishment of him and to very likely to the delight of his partner.

3. Back to sleep problems. Some people have problems in their 30's or 40's to fall asleep. Melatonin is the known hormone from the pineal gland that initiates and maintains sleep. Melatonin happens to be the human hormone that decreases first (1). Above the age of 20 to 30, melatonin production begins to decline. Look at the graph in this link. It's clear why many people benefit from a 3 mg dose of melatonin at bedtime. This could be repeated should you wake up in the middle of the night. There is no side effect, because melatonin is a hormone that the body knows. You also will not feel groggy I the morning.

4. Menopause and andropause also affect hormone production. We've already discussed the lack of testosterone in andropause. But women also need hormone replacement when they enter menopause. With the replacement they will not experience the menopausal problems like hot flashes.

In conclusion, many people are surprised by the decline in hormone production, as they get older. They should supplement with bioidentical hormones to rebalance the hormone system.

Internet reference

1. http://www.askdrray.com/wp-content/uploads/2014/02/Melatonin-More-Than-A-Sleeping-Aid.png

Chapter 27:

Hospital

Why do physicians keep some patients in hospital overnight?

The reasons for keeping a patient overnight in the hospital can be as varied as the clinical conditions.

1. If a patient took an overdose of pills or alcohol, you want to observe the vital signs and make sure the patient breathes on his/her own. By keeping the patient overnight and observe clinically the nursing staff and the doctor make sure that it is safe to send the patient home the following morning.

2. Sometimes a patient with breathing problems (like asthma) seems to be better initially after an adrenalin injection. It makes it safer to keep the patient overnight to monitor the breathing and be sure the asthma attack does not come back overnight.

3. A patient with an infection around a wound needs intravenous antibiotics to reach high antibiotic levels to kill the bacteria in the wound. Often it takes only overnight monitoring to be certain that the antibiotic works. The patient can be sent home in the morning and be brought back every 12 hours for further IV doses until it is safe

to switch to oral antibiotics when the infection is clearly controlled.

4. A psychotic patient is brought in to the emergency room. It is not quite clear whether the psychosis is due to a street drug or whether it is from a flare-up of schizophrenia. The purpose of an overnight observation is to see which course the psychosis is taking overnight. If the patient had a psychosis as a result of taking a street drug, it likely will be gone in the morning. But if it was due to a flare-up of schizophrenia, the patient will have to be hospitalized for further treatments. Drug induced psychoses usually wears off fast and the patient may be able to be sent home the following morning. Overnight admissions are done for the safety of the patient and to monitor his or her condition.

Internet reference

1. https://en.wikipedia.org/wiki/Substance-induced_psychosis

Chapter 28:

Infections

Can you turn blind from sharing your bed with your cat?

I am afraid that some people have ignored toxoplasmosis, which is a cat transmitted parasitic disease where humans are swallowing the microscopic eggs that can be in the feces of cats. Young cats (litters) have much more of these oocytes (eggs) in their feces than older cats (1).

Toxoplasmosis is still a feared disease in humans as it can indeed lead to blindness when the bugs multiply in the retina and take away vision. If diagnosed early enough, complicated regimens of antibiotics in association with frequent eye specialist exams are necessary to bring the eye involvement to a halt or else the person will turn blind (2).

When I grew up in Germany I still remember that toxoplasmosis was a relatively common cause of blindness. Keep in mind that the concentration of oocytes is highest in the litter box. It is for this reason that pregnant women should never empty the litter box of a cat, as this can lead to congenital toxoplasmosis, an often serious condition that can even lead to fetal death.

The question here is whether a cat sleeping in the same bed can transmit toxoplasmosis. The answer is "YES". You will wonder how this can be possible. It is disconcerting and very logical: the oocytes at the rear end of the cat can rub off onto the bed sheet. The human in the same bed inadvertently touches the bed sheet with their hands. Later the oocytes that are microscopic inadvertently get touched by the tongue and get swallowed. They find their way into the intestinal tract and the larvae enter the bloodstream. From there it is only a matter of time before they find the retina of both eyes.

Learn to prevent Toxoplasmosis:

1. Never touch a cat's rear end. If you stroke a cat, wash your hands right after.
2. Wear gloves when handling the litter box. Dispose of the gloves.

The key is to think prevention when you deal with cats.

Internet references

1. https://www.cdc.gov/parasites/toxoplasmosis/epi.html
2. https://www.cdc.gov/parasites/toxoplasmosis/health_professionals/index.html#tx

Why do I have a sore throat?

An acute inflammation of the pharynx (throat) is called "pharyngitis". This is either produced by a viral or bacterial infection. There may just be painful swallowing and a sore throat, but there may be a membrane in the back of the throat as a result of toxins produced by bacteria or viruses, and lymph node swelling underneath the chin. The toxins and the bacteria and viruses that multiply in the surface of the lining of the pharynx (throat) make it really inflamed and sore. Also, the tonsils can be swollen as well as the adenoids in the back of the nose and pain can radiate into your throat. The physician may want to take a throat culture, as it can be difficult to know whether your problems are related to a virus or bacterium. If something grows on the culture, it is bacterial, if there is no growth it is viral. During flu season the physician may do a nasal or throat swab for viruses to establish what kind of flu virus it is.

The organisms isolated on a bacterial culture can be group A Streptococcus, Mycoplasma pneumoniae, Chlamydia pneumoniae and on occasion even gonorrhea.

Treatment

This consists initially of penicillin V 250 mg four times daily for 10 days until the culture report comes back. This way rheumatic fever from group A Streptococcus can be avoided.

The final culture report may sway the physician to change the therapy according to the sensitivity testing.

Chapter 29:

Injuries

Eardrum injury by Q-tip

The eardrum gets perforated easily as it does not take much pressure to do this with a Q-tip. If you perforate the eardrum you will get very dizzy, there will be a piercing pain in the affected ear and your hearing on that ear will be significantly diminished. See an ENT specialist right away. If it is confirmed that you perforated the eardrum, it will likely need surgical repair. This procedure is called tympanoplasty. For this surgery a piece of your temporal muscle sheath is taken and this is used to patch the eardrum defect.

Publications of medical questions and answers in popular magazines.

mentalfloss.com: June 26, 2017

What is the Main Function of Blood?

Answer by Ray Schilling, M.D., author of "Healing Gone Wrong, Healing Done Right".

Blood has many functions.

1. Most of all, blood transports oxygen from the lungs to all the tissues by way of hemoglobin that is embedded in the red blood cells. On the way back to the heart and lungs it transports CO_2, which is exhaled by the lungs.

2. Nutrients are taken up in the capillaries of the gut, transported via the portal vein into the liver. Here many metabolic pathways are followed and the nutrients are further transported through the blood to all of the body cells.

3. Clotting factors in the plasma of the blood together with platelets contained in the blood see to it that any tiny tears or holes are immediately plugged. Blood has a certain blood pressure, so any defect cannot be tolerated or this could lead to a major bleed. It is interesting that coagulation from clotting factors/platelets and fibrinolysis are constantly balancing each other automatically.

4. Infection is being contained by white blood cells (lymphocytes for viruses, neutrophils for bacteria) on the one hand and antibodies from plasma cells on the other hand. This is quite an effective system to fight infection. Occasionally antibiotics are needed when our immune system is overwhelmed.

5. Hormones and other signalling molecules (e.g. nitric oxide) integrate the function of various organs. As long as all hormones are present and balanced we have energy and all our organs function perfectly. But when hormones are missing, we feel miserable. As we age, some hormones are not produced sufficiently. Having reviewed the literature, bioidentical hormone replacement will allow our system to get rebalanced.

6. Heat distribution and blood redistribution are other aspect of perfusion of our limbs with blood, our abdominal organs, the head and skin. After a meal the blood is rushing

to the gut and the liver as we start to digest our meal. We may get tired, because some of the blood from the brain gets pulled away to the stomach, small intestine and the liver. On a hot day our skin veins open up wide, we sweat and lose some of our body heat through our skin. It's the body's way to keep us cool inside.

7. There is one aspect that seems to be out of our control. When we get excited or a person is extremely shy, the head, neck, and the ears will turn red. This is out of our control. Some people have this more than others and some don't have it at all. It comes from dilated skin blood vessels. When they dilate, blood rushes into that region giving your skin a reddened appearance.

How dangerous is it to bite your tongue?

I have not seen anybody die from it. I have stitched up tongue lacerations in the Emergency Room of the local hospital. Tongue lacerations bleed first, but then they stop and bleed a bit again. Most people use common sense and get checked out at a hospital or walk-in clinic, especially if the wound is larger and does not stop bleeding. I never heard of anyone bleeding to death. This sounds highly unusual. A sensationalist story on TV would sound like this: "Patient bled to death after biting his tongue", or maybe Hollywood would be interested to film a horror movie? By the way: any laceration in the mouth tends to heal extremely fast on its own. This should reassure you!

Chapter 30:

Keeping Your Brain Healthy

Foods for brain health

The fact that the type of diet you eat has a lot to do with your brain health keeps popping up in the medical literature, and 2015 has not been any exception.

1. The Mediterranean diet in particular has been shown to have very positive effects on postponing Alzheimer's disease by as much as 5 years (1).

2. A clinical study on 674 elderly patients (mean age 80.1 years) without dementia, was published in the journal "Neurology". It examined the question whether adherence to the Mediterranean diet would affect the degree of brain atrophy, which in turn is known to correlate with the onset of Alzheimer's disease. The findings were interesting: a high adherence to the Mediterranean diet led to a higher total brain volume, total grey matter volume and total white matter volume as measured with high-resolution structural MRI scans. Lower meat intake led to higher brain volume and more fish intake caused the mean cortical thickness of the brain to increase. Parts of the brain that are affected in Alzheimer's patients with atrophy like the cingulate cortex, parietal lobe, temporal lobe, and hippocampus showed

good volumes with the MRI scans when patients adhered to the Mediterranean diet. These volumes started to shrink when the diet was poor.

3. Those who adhered to the Mediterranean diet have brains that on MRI scan look 5 years younger and are much less likely to get affected by Alzheimer's disease (2). Physicians have known for a long time that people, who eat a healthy diet, exercise regularly, don't smoke and who keep mentally stimulated will generally have healthier brains than people who don't do these things.

4. What is the Mediterranean diet? It involves eating meals that are made up of plants: vegetables, fruit, cereals, beans and nuts. You can eat fish and poultry twice per week. You cut down the amount of meat and dairy you eat, but you can have a glass of wine per day, if you like. Butter is not used for cooking, but olive oil is used instead. Here is more information of what is included in the Mediterranean diet. Because there is less fat and less high glycemic index carbs in this diet, it is also a diet that lends itself for weight management (3). You shed a few pounds and reach your ideal body mass index without paying much attention to this. Apart from the Mediterranean diet another diet, called the MIND diet has also been shown to prevent brain atrophy (4). This diet is a combination of the DASH diet that was developed for controlling high blood pressure and the Mediterranean diet.

5. The Mediterranean diet makes you live longer and healthier. The Nurses' Health Study that has been going on since 1976 showed that telomeres, the caps on chromosomes, were getting shorter in nurses who lived on junk foods, but surprisingly nurses on the Mediterranean diet preserved their telomeres (5). Longer telomeres are associated with slower aging. And people with longer telomeres reach an older age without diseases like heart attacks, liver disease or cancer.

6. Exercise combined with the Mediterranean diet. It is not a good idea to just rely on a healthy diet, like the Mediterranean diet to prevent heart attacks, strokes and other diseases. You need regular exercise as the other ingredient to keep you well. When you combine exercise with a healthy diet your abdominal girth shrinks as this study showed (6).

Another study showed that when a Mediterranean type diet is combined with regular exercise, adult onset diabetes occurrence could be reduced by 28-59% (7).

This is quite a significant effect of two simple interventions: a healthy diet and regular exercise. Other literature has shown that Alzheimer's disease is more common in diabetics. In those who do not have diabetes, the frequency of Alzheimer's disease is much less common.

Internet references

1. http://www.cnn.com/2015/10/21/health/mediterranean-diet-healthier-brain/index.html
2. http://n.neurology.org/content/early/2015/10/21/WNL.0000000000002121
3. https://www.cdc.gov/nccdphp/dnpa/nutrition/pdf/rtp_practitioner_10_07.pdf
4. https://www.rush.edu/news/press-releases/new-mind-diet-may-significantly-protect-against-alzheimers-disease
5. http://www.cnn.com/2014/12/03/health/mediterranean-diet-longevity/
6. https://www.ncbi.nlm.nih.gov/pubmed/26493478
7. https://www.ncbi.nlm.nih.gov/pubmed/20337844

Chapter 31:

Life Expectancy

What is the theoretical life expectancy of humans?

Right now the average lifespan in industrial countries is around 80 to 84 years. But this is because the majority of people do not take good care of themselves. Some people with longevity genes make it to about 120 years.
The limiting factors are the telomere lengths of your chromosomes. Next the DNA within the mitochondria is very vulnerable to DNA breaks or mutations. This robs you of the energy providing subunits within each cell. Without energy there is no life.
How can people take care of themselves? Quit smoking, if you do, as smoking is an aging substance. Avoid extra sugar intake. Limit refined carb intake and instead eat complex carbs like vegetables and fruit. Exercise regularly. Eat a balanced diet like the Mediterranean diet. This has been shown to be anti-inflammatory and many life-shortening illnesses are due to chronic inflammation. Take some vitamins and supplements like vitamin D3, fish oil, selenium, zinc, magnesium, Co-Q 10 and quercetin. Make sure you get enough sleep and do not forget activities that contribute to relaxation to counter stress.

As you age your hormone glands will produce less and less hormones. Find an anti-aging physician or naturopathic physician who understands bioidentical hormone replacement. Have your hormones measured and only replace what is missing. Repeat hormone tests to document that the replacement is working. This includes human growth hormone replacement, if tests show that it is missing.

Using this approach more people could reach an age of 120 years. They certainly can live longer than they do now.

More info on this topic here (1).

Internet reference

1. http://www.askdrray.com/life-extended-by-several-decades/

Publications of medical questions and answers in popular magazines.

apple.news: Aug. 17, 2017

The Tips of Your Chromosomes Can Tell Doctors About Your Health

Answer by Ray Schilling, M.D., author of "Healing Gone Wrong, Healing Done Right".

The end caps of chromosomes are called telomeres. At the 22nd Annual World Congress on Anti-Aging Medicine in Las Vegas (Dec.10 to 14, 2014) stem cells, telomeres, hormones and lifestyle were the highlights of that year's conference.

Dr. Sandy Chang gave a talk about "Telomere measurement as a diagnostic test in cardiovascular and age-related disease". He pointed out that there is a large body of literature showing that telomere length is directly related to health (1).

The shorter the telomeres are, the higher is the probability to experience problems: early menopause, infertility, diabetes, wrinkles, arthritis, osteoporosis, cardiovascular disease, Alzheimer's, Parkinson's, dementia, cancer, stress, a lack of stem cells (2).

These are a number of factors that shorten telomeres: stress, poor diet, smoking, obesity, chronic inflammatory diseases, metabolic disorders like diabetes, over consumption of alcohol and lack of sleep.

Dr. Chang mentioned that there is a whole host of factors that can elongate telomeres by stimulating telomerase. It has been shown in humans that increased physical activity elongated telomeres. So did vitamin C, E and vitamin D3 supplementation, resveratrol, a Mediterranean diet and marine omega-3 fatty acid supplementation. In addition higher fiber intake, bioidentical estrogen in women and testosterone in men, relaxation techniques like yoga and meditation are also elongating telomeres.

Other speakers also talked about telomeres: Dr. Al Sears' talk was entitled: "Telo-Nutritioneering: The latest generation of telomere modulators". He mentioned that in his research he has identified at least 123 nutrients, vitamins and natural compounds that will elongate telomeres, often by stimulating telomerase. Vitamin C will significantly delay shortening of telomeres, which translates into delayed aging. In addition, vitamin C has recently been shown to stimulate telomerase activity in certain stem cells. There is an herb, called Silymarin extract, which was recently found to increase telomerase activity threefold. N-acetyl cysteine is a building block for glutathione, a powerful anti-oxidant. In addition, it has been shown to turn on the human telomerase gene. Other telomerase stimulators are green tea extract, ginkgo biloba, gamma tocotrienol (one of the components of the vitamin E group), vitamin D3 and folic acid.

Internet references

1. https://en.wikipedia.org/wiki/Telomere
2. http://www.bmj.com/content/349/bmj.g4227

What is the life expectancy for humans in this day and age?

1. Most anti-aging experts from the A4M say that right now our life expectancy limit would be at 115 to 120 years. But other A4M members say that it may be at 130 to 135 years. Right now the average life expectancy is about 80 years.

2. If you add multiple vitamin and trace minerals, you can add 9.8 years to the baseline of 80 years. The reason is that multiple vitamins have been shown to elongate your telomeres by 5.1% (page 283 of Ref. 1), which translates into 9.8 years longer life.

3. If you add bioidentical hormone replacement you can add 15 years of good life. This brings you to 104.8 years (80+9.8+15).

4. If growth hormone deficiency is present as evidenced by low IGF-1 blood levels or low overnight urine collection (human growth hormone metabolites), this needs to be replaced with daily 0.1mg to 0.2mg of human growth hormone by skin injections at bedtime. A tiny insulin-syringe like injection needle is used for this. Those who do this have a 26.5-year average addition of healthy life. This is how powerful human growth hormone is when the dosage is administered appropriately (page 165 of Ref.1). Human growth hormone is particularly important in aging people. The total now is 131.3 years. (80+9.8+15+26.5).

Not everybody will want to shoulder the cost of human growth hormone. But others may be eligible with their health plans to get coverage as it is a true hormone deficiency in many aging people, but under diagnosed. This is how science has broken down the factors that increase life expectancy. Another factor is longevity as a family trait.

Book reference

Ref.1: Dr. Ray Schilling, 2016: "Healing Gone Wrong - Healing Done Right", Amazon 2016.
https://www.amazon.com/gp/product/1523700904

What can be done so we can live forever?

For starters let's get realistic. Nobody lives forever! The fact is that there are several layers that can help to prolong your life. All of the factors that will follow have in common that they want to preserve your life as it is right now. This means your mitochondrial function, your DNA, your telomeres all need to be preserved. Let me get into specifics (4 points). But after that I will come to a conclusion.

1. Telomeres and the biology of aging

In one study the telomere length at the age of 100 was only 40% compared to the age of 20. Now we are learning that telomeres can be lengthened by healthy lifestyles. It has been shown in humans that increased physical activity elongated telomeres. So did vitamin C, E, vitamin D3 supplementation and resveratrol. A Mediterranean diet and marine omega-3 fatty acid supplementation elongate telomeres as well. In addition higher fiber intake, bioidentical estrogen in women and testosterone in men have been shown to elongate telomeres. Finally, relaxation techniques like yoga and meditation are also elongating telomeres.

2. Mitochondria and the biology of aging

Mitochondria can be preserved through exercise, CoQ-10 supplementation and caloric restriction (1).
This overcomes a lack of energy and strengthens your muscles including the heart. As Dr. Whitaker has shown in this link, it is simple. Eat less, exercise more and take nutritional supplements.

3. Hormone deficiencies and the biology of aging

Another factor of aging is hormone deficiency in general and growth hormone (GH) deficiency in particular. In the past it was thought that growth hormone was only important for bone growth in children and young teenagers. However, more research revealed that it has also an important maintenance function. This maintenance concerns our muscles including the heart and to preserve our brain. Here is a review article about human growth hormone deficiency that may be mind-blowing to you (2).
When people age, they lose GH production, putting them at a considerable risk to get heart attacks and strokes. But they are also at a higher risk of serious falls due to muscle weakness and balance problems. When the doctor detects low IGF-1 levels in the blood this is a sign of GH deficiency. This has to be confirmed by low GH metabolites in a 24-hour urine sample.
When this is also showing GH deficiency, the time has come to do daily GH injections with human GH. This can be done using a similar pen that is used for insulin injections. The dosage is only between 0.1 mg and 0.3 mg per day, given before bedtime. This is remarkably effective not only for heart attack and stroke prevention, but also to treat muscle weakness. In addition it treats lack of mental clarity and increases general well being. Patients report that their

joint and muscle aches disappear. They can engage in physical activities again. But GH is not the only hormone that needs to be observed and when low be replaced by nature-identical hormones (3).

4. DNA of our cells

The big question is how do we preserve DNA against damage from the everyday metabolism by-products and ionizing radiation from space? There are many open questions. Our DNA does not sit still, it constantly moves, genes are activated and suppressed, and in this process we lose cancer suppressor genes causing cancer that eventually would kill us. Our scientists today are smart, but they are not that smart that they would know all the future research results they have not yet detected.

Conclusion

At the 23rd Annual World Congress on Anti-Aging Medicine on Dec. 13, 2015 in Las Vegas the endocrinologist, Dr. Thierry Hertoghe from Belgium gave a talk about "How to extend the human lifespan by 40 years". It does sound optimistic, and here are his explanations.

He said that bioidentical hormone replacement could add 15 years of life. Organ transplants, if necessary, telomerase activators and stem cell therapy can add another 25 years of life expectancy to a total of 40 years. He felt that there is a limit of about 120 to 125 years of life expectancy. I have blogged on this here: life extended by several decades (4).

I am afraid at the present time we are limited to a possible life extension "only" until about age 120 to 125. As a result the "living forever" concept is simply not in the cards, unless you find a way to preserve DNA from damages. The only way nature has done this since its existence is by rejuvenation through eggs and sperms creating new life.

For now we can enjoy life for several decades longer than our forefathers. This is not bad, and we have every reason to enjoy this fact.

More info about biology of aging here (5).

Internet references

1. https://www.drwhitaker.com/3-ways-to-tune-up-your-mitochondria-and-enhance-energy/
2. https://www.ncbi.nlm.nih.gov/pmc/articles/PMC3183535/
3. http://www.askdrray.com/effects-of-hormones-on-the-heart/
4. http://www.askdrray.com/life-extended-by-several-decades/
5. http://nethealthbook.com/news/the-biology-of-aging/

How come it is impossible to extend the human lifespan beyond a certain limit?

It is possible to extend human life up to about 120 to 125 years.

But it is difficult to help people to live beyond this limit, as our DNA gets so damaged in time that cell function becomes impossible. The telomeres are also shortened to the point where they will not support further cell divisions. Finally, our mitochondria, the power source within our cells are suffering irreparable damage. And without energy we cannot live.

This is all based on our present knowledge of cell functioning. Future basic research into these problems may come up with newer insights. But presently these limits are what keep us from reaching an age beyond 120 or 125 years.

Chapter 32:

Lifestyle Habits

Can good habits change your life completely?

Here is what I did in the last few years.

1. I cut out wheat and wheat products since 2001 as prevention against leaky gut syndrome and autoimmune diseases.

2. I started exercising regularly. My muscles are stronger. I have more endurance. I feel more energetic, which helps me to have sustained energy with any physical activity, going to the gym as well as having fun ballroom and Latin dancing; (my wife does the same).

3. I cut out all sugar, honey and starchy foods like bread, pasta, and white rice since 2001. This allows me to have excellent LDL values and HDL values. I did a VAP tests and had excellent values there.

I also had a carotid intima scan, which essentially showed no hardening of the arteries.

4. I retired when I was 65 rather than wait until age 67 or later. This was the best thing in my life, but I am still busy writing blogs, books and answering medical questions wherever I can.

5. Change has kept me on my toes. I enjoy doing handiwork around the house.

6. Change started early on: I moved from Germany to Canada, and even though not all changes are easy, it is my firm believe that they help us to keep flexible, and flexibility helps to slow down aging.

Do I think these facts have changed my life completely? Yes, I do. In the meantime I have switched from practicing medicine to writing about medicine. Knowing that people like you read my books and blogs, and get some health benefits from this material for themselves, is rewarding for me!

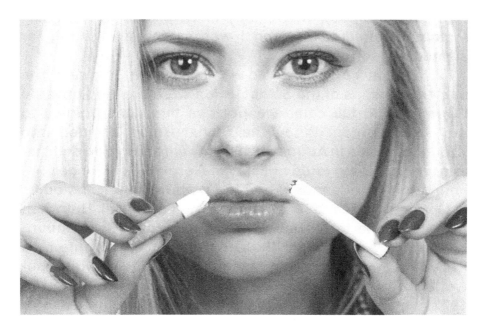

Internet reference

1. http://www.medfusion.net/templates/groups/7241/12677/VAP.pdf

How did key happenings in your life change your life direction?

Life is full of consequences. But whatever is thrown at you by fate can turn into a learning experience that gives you a chance to change in which direction you want to go. Here are a couple of key experiences that shaped my life:

1. My first experience was Waldorf School at the age of 7 years. It id not work for me! After one year of suffering through this I complained to my mother that I was still only drawing pictures of a table, but nobody taught me how to spell "table". I told her that I wanted to go to a regular elementary school, where they learn proper spelling. My mother listened to me and I was switched to a regular elementary school.

2. We grew up in the cold war in Western Germany. The nuclear missiles of the Soviet Union were pointing towards Germany and the same weapons of the Allies pointed to the Soviet Union. When the Soviet Union invaded into Czechoslovakia in August of 1968 my wife and I decided that this was it (1).We would not stay in Germany any longer, but immigrate into Canada. I had to finish my medical studies in Germany first and finish my internship as well. But when this was done in the fall of 1972, we moved to a suburb of Toronto. I worked for the Ontario Cancer Institute as a PhD student. In case the cancer research idea would not work out I took the ECFMG exam in Munich in spring of 1972, which qualified me to work as an intern in the US or in Canada. I was now 27 years old.

3. My mother had died of colon cancer in 1980. I felt helpless, but had a dream of studying medicine and curing cancer. This did not happen. But what happened was that I started a job as a PhD student at the Ontario Cancer Institute (now called Princess Margaret Cancer Centre) doing cancer research in October of 1972. After

three publications I talked to a guy who had finished his PhD. He looked all over Canada and could not find a job in cancer research. So he was driving a taxi in Montreal. I was slaving away long hours on a small cancer research stipend, although I was a fully trained physician abroad with the prospect of driving a taxi as an MD, PhD. My wife and I had some deep discussions about that. If you want to read more about my cancer research experience, here is a blog that I wrote (2).At the end I decided to walk away from a 75% completed PhD and instead started an internship at McMaster University. I went through the regulations to become a practicing physician in Canada. At the end of cancer research I was 30 years old.

4. Snowstorm in 1977: what does a snowstorm of 3 feet have to do with life decisions? This snowstorm in Hamilton/Ont. killed several people and I came home after work at a university hospital on a snowmobile of a neighbor. I had to abandon my car as everybody was stuck. My wife and I had another long talk and decided that we would move west where the climate was milder. This actually happened in the summer of 1978 after I had passed the Canadian LMCC, the Canadian licensing exam. I was now finished with my training and found work as a second physician in an office in Langley, a suburb of Vancouver, BC. This was what I wanted: practice medicine in a general practice setting. I also treated a lot of cancer patients, so the experience at the Ontario Cancer Institute was not for nothing. Early cancer detection and early treatment was the motto. When we moved to Langley I was 33 years old.

5. In the last years of general practice (I did this for 16 years) I felt that being on call at night and doing night time deliveries was just too much in addition to the regular busy life in general practice. I decided it was time for a change again. I had a phone call from one of the Medical Advisors of WCB regarding one of my patients who were laid off after a

work injury. I asked this colleague what it was like working for WCB. He painted a picture of regulated work hours, 3 weeks of paid holidays initially, going up to 5 weeks of paid holidays after a few years. Would I like to join? They were in need of more Medical Advisors. A few weeks later I sold my practice and joined WCB in October of 1994. I was 49 years old. I moved to the interior of British Columbia where I practiced as a Medical Advisor of WCB (later called WorkSafe BC) for another 16 years until my retirement in 2010, at which time I was 65 years old. I am now 73 years, maintain two medical websites since 2002 and have written 4 books (you are reading my 4th one right now).

Internet references

1. http://www.history.com/this-day-in-history/soviets-invade-czechoslovakia
2. http://www.askdrray.com/my-experience-with-cancer-research/

What things do I need to do every day to get the best out of life?

1. It helps to more or less have a sleep/wake rhythm, meaning that you go to bed between 10 and 11 PM and wake up after 7 to 8 hours of sleep. Your room needs to be dark so that your diurnal hormone rhythm resets itself automatically every night while you sleep. Your regular sleep rhythm will ensure that you have lots of energy the following day.

2. Eating healthy year-in and year-out is a given as far as I am concerned. Read my answer to this question under "Diet": What are some key facts about healthy food consumption? I am explaining there what to eat and what to avoid.

But many people find this a challenge. At home I can buy organic food and my wife can cook or prepare it (I can too, but she is better at it). We attend the Anti-Aging Conferences in Las Vegas regularly that take place in the middle of December every year. Eating in Las Vegas can be a challenge. We were lucky that in many American cities and towns there are health food stores and grocery chains that sell wholesome, organic foods and even have a cafeteria-style self-serve section. One of the outlets of such a chain is present in Las Vegas where we could eat lunch or dinner. The rest of the time we were able to prepare our own organic food we had bought there, as our condo where we stayed had a kitchen facility. The healthier you live, the more energy you have and the longer you will live as we learnt again at the A4M (American Academy of Anti-Aging Medicine) conference.

3. Now you have time to do what you may have to do, like working, studying etc. I leave this section up to you to fill in. There is one important point: in our everyday life we are bombarded with challenges, and they can be a source of stress. It is extremely important to manage stress situations. Stress can kill! By the way, anger can also throw a monkey wrench into our emotional and physical health!

4. After work or during your day activities, if you are retired, you should make time for a 1-hour workout. The problem in our society is that we tend to be rather sessile during section 3 (working, studying, leisure activities). In the so-called blue-zone societies centenarians were found to be very active people moving all day long: Can 'Blue Zones' help turn back the biological clock (1)?

But we can still live longer than the average person, if we keep ourselves fit in a gym. It will keep your LDL cholesterol low, your HDL cholesterol high and your triglycerides low. The end result: no heart attacks and strokes, even less cancer and Alzheimer's disease. You end up with a longer life without disabilities.

5. Socializing: you need real person interaction. Texting on the phone or sitting around and connecting on social media does not do it! Talking to others who are on a similar wavelength as you are of help to keep you going. But you also need to come to terms regarding human sexuality. It is a source of constant energy for both partners. Long-term studies have shown that stable relationships add 3 years of life expectancy over a lifetime for both partners.

6. Hobbies can be a source of satisfaction and fun, which would give you extra energy and enjoyment. Sports activities, when not overdone, give you exercise and satisfaction. Meditation, yoga and self-hypnosis are activities that can help you with relaxation and are great helpers in stress management.

Conclusion

I outlined some of my thoughts that may help you to sort out what to do to have a good life. Listen around; the input of friends can be very valuable! But most of all think for yourself what is the best mix for you.

Internet reference

1. http://www.npr.org/templates/story/story.php?storyId=91285403

Can smoking and drinking ruin my health?

Smoking is the leading cause of preventable death: 1 in 5 deaths in the US are due to smoking. Who smokes in the US (1)?

You would never know that this is so, because smoking is a silent killer. It gets you hooked, then you enjoy it for years and years. When you quit and think you got away with it, this previous habit can still be a killer: pancreatic cancer, lung cancer, stomach cancer, and chronic obstructive lung disease are some of the deadly consequences. Here are the effects of cigarette smoke on your body (2):

As this link shows, various parts of the body react differently to these chemicals. Here is a rundown of diseases caused by smoking cigarettes.

1. Lung cancer: This is the most common cause of death in women who smoke, more common now than breast cancer. 90% of lung cancers in women are due to smoking. The same was true in males, but as a group they now smoke less than in the past.

2. Other cancers: cervical cancer, kidney cancer, pancreatic cancer, bladder, esophageal, stomach, laryngeal, oral, and throat cancers are all caused by smoking. Recently acute myeloid leukemia, a cancer of the bone marrow has been added to the list of smoking related cancers.

3. Abdominal aortic aneurysm: As cigarette smoke destroys elastic tissue, it is no wonder that the loss of support of the wall of the aortic artery leads to the development of large pouches, which eventually rupture with a high mortality rate due to massive blood loss.

4. Infections of lungs and gums: Smokers are prone to infections of the lungs (pneumonia) and of the gums (periodontitis).

5. Chronic lung diseases: emphysema, chronic bronchitis, asthma.

6. Cataracts: lack of perfusion of the lens leads to premature cataract formation.

7. Coronary heart disease: hardening of the coronary arteries, which leads to heart attacks, is very common in smokers.

8. Reproduction: reduced fertility in mothers, premature rupture of membranes with prematurely born babies; low

birth weight; all this leads to higher infant mortality. Sudden infant death syndrome is found more frequently in children of smoking moms.

9. Intermittent claudication: after decades of smoking the larger arteries in the legs are hardening, and not enough oxygen reaches the muscles to walk causing intermittent pausing to recover from the muscle aches. If it is feasible a cardiovascular surgeon may be able to do a bypass surgery to rescue the legs, often though this is not feasible and the patients lower legs or an entire lower limb may have to be amputated.

10. Others: osteoporosis is more common in smokers; poor eye sight develops due to age-related macular degeneration that sets in earlier and due to tobacco amblyopia, a toxic effect from tobacco on the optic nerve; hypothyroidism is aggravated by smoking, and menopause occurs earlier.

Conclusion

You are in control of your destiny. Don't underestimate the viciousness of cigarette smoke. Eventually it gets you. Don't become a statistic; quit smoking instead, and do it now!

Internet references

1. http://money.cnn.com/infographic/news/who-smokes-in-the-us/?hpt=hp_t3
2. http://www.therapy-store.com/smoking/women__tobacco.htm

Do exercise and diet influence your life expectancy?

1. The right diet will make sure food intake is anti-inflammatory. For instance, the Mediterranean diet and the

DASH diet are anti-inflammatory diets. When you don't have chronic inflammation you will stay healthier for longer.

2. Regular exercise keeps your circulation going, maintains your cardiovascular fitness, improves your immune system, keeps your muscles in good shape and elongates your telomeres. This has been shown to be associated with longevity and a lack of Alzheimer's disease.

3. But if you are serious about extending your lifespan, you need a couple of more ingredients. As you age, you must ask your doctor, anti-aging physician or naturopath to measure your hormones. As we age we lose thyroid hormones, sex hormones, melatonin, DHA and human growth hormone. Any deficiencies in these likely have to be replaced and monitored (1).

4. We also know that relaxation methods like yoga, Tai Chi, meditation or self-hypnosis lead to anti-inflammatory markers in the blood stream. The suppression of any inflammation is known to prevent heart attacks, strokes, diabetes and even Alzheimer's disease. The end result is an extension of your lifespan: relaxation reduces inflammation (2).

Internet references

1. http://www.askdrray.com/bioidentical-hormone-replacement-2/
2. http://www.askdrray.com/relaxation-reduces-inflammation/

Health impact of smoking cigarettes and drinking alcohol

1. Drinking alcohol is different than smoking is for getting lung cancer. But in a strange way the two are related. Because there is a relationship between cigarettes smoked and getting lung cancer. At the same time it also causes

heart attacks and strokes as well as pancreatic cancer and cancer of the esophagus.

2. Now when you look at the amount of alcohol consumed and what disease of the liver develops in time, you notice that the first disease that occurs is liver cirrhosis. This is a fibrotic degeneration of the liver tissue. When you continue to drink alcoholic beverages, you start getting cancer cells and eventually that is what can kill you.

3. Both cigarette smoke and alcohol are cell poisons. It is not surprising that smoking can cause lung cancer and consumption of regular high amounts of alcohol can cause liver cancer.

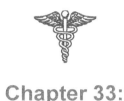

Chapter 33:

Pain

Pain relief for a headache or other pain: Aleve, Advil or Tylenol?

Tylenol is the best to use. The other two are anti-inflammatories. Many people are not aware that Advil and all the other anti-inflammatories like ASA and NSAIDs (which includes Aleve) shorten telomeres. Telomeres, the caps of chromosomes are important for a long life. Telomeres can also be shortened by chronic stress and a chronic lack of sleep. We need long telomeres for a long life!

Publications of medical questions and answers in popular magazines.

Apple.news: June 15, 2017

Why Our Bodies Ache as We Age and How We Can Prevent It

Answer by Ray Schilling, M.D., author of "Healing Gone Wrong, Healing Done Right".

Why does our body hurt when we get old?

For many people osteoarthritis can lead to chronic pain. When aging joints lose the hyaline cartilage coating, eventually bone rubs on bone. Many people think that they need to accept this pain. Conservative physicians play into that passive thinking. They wait until the pain is so excruciating and then they refer you to an orthopedic surgeon for a total hip or knee replacement.

However, there is an alternative: prolotherapy, platelet-rich plasma (PRP) or stem cell therapy. These are newer methods that work quite well, but are often ignored by conventional physicians. If they are applied, pain often disappears and mobility returns. Patients who do these therapies end up cancelling their appointments for total joint replacement. Besides, these surgeries often fail to give the promised relief.

Hormone deficiencies are also often leading to muscle aches and pains. A lack of testosterone can do this to a male (andropause); a lack of estrogen and progesterone to a female (menopause).

Low thyroid levels will rob you of energy, make you depressed and give you aching muscles.

When you look after all of these hormones (bioidentical hormone replacement), you may still have achy muscles and joints from human growth hormone (HGH) deficiency, which can be diagnosed by a blood test (IGF-1) and an expensive overnight urine HGH metabolite test. When this is replaced with daily bedtime needles of HGH (low dose) similar to insulin injections, your energy can come back and the achy muscles disappear for good and your thinking sharpens.

You need to exercise daily to keep your muscles and joints in good order. You need to follow a sensible diet like the Mediterranean diet. Your body needs vegetables and salads. You also need omega-3 fatty acid supplements and a good dose of vitamin D3.

You don't need to hurt when you get old. But if you hurt, you must think about all of your options. Think about seeing other health professionals like a naturopathic physician, an integrative medicine doctor or a regenerative medicine doctor. The field of medicine is expanding outside of conventional medicine. Cover the whole arena, if you need help. Otherwise do your part in keeping yourself young!

Chapter 34:

Parenting

Has the old slogan "tough love" backfired?

"Tough love" was a slogan in the 1970's and 1980's (1). The thought was to let the child feel the consequences of their actions and hopefully they would come around as decent people when they grow up. The problem with that is that it could become a blueprint for revenge thinking and even abuse. And the child may stay "tough" and cause problems for society by turning into an abusive adult.

It still is difficult today to raise kids as it always has been in the past. But a parent must love a child to give the child a basic parent/child relationship where it can grow into a loving adult.

In my opinion the old "tough love" idea has backfired.

Internet reference

1. https://en.wikipedia.org/wiki/Tough_love

Chapter 35:

Pregnancy

I am pregnant and following my first ultrasound scan I was told that my baby is not healthy. I was advised to abort. What should I do?

Ask questions why your baby is not healthy. Is there an abnormality? Is there a genetic defect? It would help to have either an amniocentesis or chorionic villi sampling done to determine the karyotype (1).

Typically this is done around 12 to 13 weeks. After these investigations are done, the results should be discussed between you, your husband and the specialist. Ask what other people did who were in the same situation as you are in now.

Internet reference

1. https://en.wikipedia.org/wiki/Chorionic_villus_sampling

How can a female get pregnant?

1. She has to have unprotected sex with a male, and he needs to have an orgasm into her vagina. Pregnancy can

also occur if she has sex and the method of "pulling out" is used. There may be viable sperm, and this does not work as a form of birth control.

2. She should be around the time of her ovulation. This gives the sperm that will crawl up into her tubes the highest probability of meeting and penetrating the egg that is released. Only ONE sperm will be declared the winner.

3. She has started the pregnancy. Of course there have to be the first few cell divisions and implantation into the uterine wall. The placenta needs to grow, and pregnancy needs to get across the first critical 12 to 13 weeks to be firmly established.

4. Best age for successful pregnancy. My experience with the outcome of pregnancies in my own patient load was that women between the ages of 20 and 30 had the easiest deliveries. But there are always possible exceptions. An older woman can have an easy delivery while another woman at that age may have all kinds of complications. There are also more problems with young women at age 17 to 19. Yet, as is always the case, there can be exceptions where pregnancy is uneventful and delivery just fine.

Overall my impression is that age 20 to 30 is best and always has been best for getting babies for women. Unfortunately this does not always go too well with higher education and delayed plans for settling down. But biological facts are difficult to argue with.

Chapter 36:

Prostate Cancer

How dangerous is prostate cancer? Does it kill you?

   1. Yes, prostate cancer kills like any other cancer. There are 4 stages of prostate cancer where specialists determine how far spread the cancer is when they diagnose prostate cancer. Below I am presenting survival statistics based on thousands of actual patients. If the cancer is early, it looks like prostate cancer would be harmless. Stage A prostate cancer has survival rates of 100% after 5 years and 97% after 10 years. But, if you leave this cancer alone, then stage D may develop after a few more years. Now the survival rates are only 29% after 5 years and 0% after 10 years of follow-up.

   2. Staging of prostate cancer is as important as in other cancers. It allows the physician to assess at which level the cancer is at the time of diagnosis. This is called staging. It might involve some X rays, perhaps a bone scan and more blood tests such as an acid phosphatase, which correlates well with the presence of metastases. A transrectal ultrasound (TRUS) and a TRUS guided prostate biopsy in 6 different areas of the prostate would also be

required. The prostate biopsy material can be analyzed by the pathologist according to how well differentiated the cells look under the microscope. A comparison is made between the grading of the normal looking cells and the worst looking prostate cancer cells in the biopsy specimens. These scores are added and a Gleason score is obtained. The higher the number, the more aggressive the cancer cells are believed to be. Mostly scores are in the 6 to 7 (out of 10) Gleason score category. An 8 (out of 10) score would be a more aggressive cancer.

3. Finally the doctor may want to employ a CT or MRI scan to delineate any involvement of the cancer outside the prostatic capsule. It helps with accurate staging.

The following stages have conventionally been used:

Staging of Prostate Cancer (Whitmore-Jewett Staging)

Stage:

A: Positive PSA and confirmed by biopsy, confined to one lobe, is clinically not visible by imaging techniques or exam

B: Is clinically palpable by rectal exam; visible on TRUS, subclasses confined to one or both lobes

C: Extends through prostatic capsule with local regional metastases, sometimes with seminal vesicle invasion

D: Prostate is fixed due to extensive invasion of adjacent structures including pelvic bone, may also have distant metastases

The significance of this staging procedure becomes evident when we look at the cancer survival rates (see below).

Prostate cancer survival

Stage	5-year survival	10-year survival
A:	100%	97%
B:	89%	71%
C:	80%	66%
D:	29%	0%

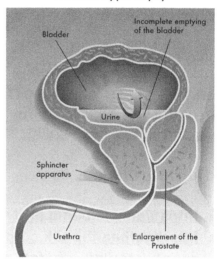

It is very clear from these statistics and the knowledge of the biology of prostate cancer that there is no such thing as a "clinically unimportant" prostate cancer. If the early cancer is missed (stage A or B), it progresses relentlessly into stage C or D and kills the patient. The TNM staging system is an alternative staging system and was developed by the American Joint Committee on Cancer. Here is a link to the TNM staging system for prostate cancer (1).

This table also tells that as long as the patient has a localized prostate cancer (stage A), there is hope for long-term survival. For the first time in millenniums with the help of the PSA test in combination with a rectal examination we have the tools of changing history. With prostate cancer we are at a similar point in time where we were with cervical cancer cure rates in women in the 1960's and 1970's. Every educated woman in the world knows that a yearly Pap test and pelvic examination can prevent cancer of the cervix and ovarian cancer. Every man from now on will accept that he has a responsibility to prevent prostate cancer.

This info was first published here (2).

I also published a book on prostate cancer in 2017 (Ref. 1).

Book reference

Ref. 1: Dr. Ray Schilling, 2017: "Prostate Cancer Unmasked": https://www.amazon.com/Prostate-Cancer-Unmasked-Ray-Schilling/dp/1542880661

Internet references

1. https://en.wikipedia.org/wiki/Prostate_cancer_staging
2. http://nethealthbook.com/cancer-overview/prostate-cancer/staging-prostate-cancer/

Chapter 37:

Schizophrenia

What complementary approach may help a patient with schizophrenia?

Many patients with schizophrenia have a methylation defect, which is a genetic enzymatic defect in one or more enzymes that methylate various brain hormones: defects in the methylation pathways (1).

Methylation defects and vitamin supplementation

People with a methylation defect are more prone to diverse diseases like autism, depression, anxiety, schizophrenia, adrenal dysfunction, addiction, cancer, allergies, immune weakness, diabetes etc.

Here is a list of the methylation pathway vitamins and trace elements important for those who are born into families where mental illness or diabetes is frequent, as they are the ones who often have methylation defects, many of which can be corrected (Ref.1).

• Vitamin B2/riboflavin: Riboflavin is used for neonatal jaundice as part of phototherapy (2).

• Some adult patients experience relief from migraines.

- **Vitamin B6/pyridoxine:** Pyridoxal phosphate is a co-factor of many enzymatic reactions in amino acid, glucose and lipid metabolism (3).
- **Vitamin B12/methylcobalamin:** Vitamin B12 is essential for your nerve function and bone marrow function or severe anemia follows (4).

It gives you energy and keeps you normal, but it is not a cure all. Sometimes in older patients absorption is a problem, but B12 injections every couple of months can easily overcome this.

- **Folate (from food or folic acid):** Research about neural tube defects (spina bifida) in the baby of a folate deficient mother led to the discovery of folic acid (5). Heavy smokers and drinkers can get folate deficient. Folate is needed in DNA synthesis.
- **Magnesium:** Magnesium is involved in more than 300 biochemical reactions within the body (6).
- It helps with asthma, bone heath, muscle pain and prevents heart attacks. It also cures psychiatric disease like anxiety and agitation. Magnesium is a co-factor for many enzymes reactions.
- **Zinc:** Because zinc is an essential trace element, it is involved in many organ systems and zinc is used for many health problems (7).
- People may have heard that zinc is an important supplement in male infertility and erectile dysfunction. But it is also needed as a supplement in diabetes, high blood pressure, psoriasis, macular degeneration and night blindness. Zinc is a natural opponent of copper meaning that when zinc is low, copper levels in the blood are often high. This constellation can cause insomnia (8).

Conclusion

It is best to work with a physician trained in ortho-molecular medicine to sort out any metabolic defects. This requires a few special blood tests. But the above-mentioned supplements can make a significant improvement of the schizophrenic condition. The patient may still require antipsychotic medicine on top of that, but likely much less to control the symptoms.

Book Reference

Ref.1: William J. Walsh, PhD: "Nutrient Power. Heal your biochemistry and heal your brain". Skyhorse Publishing, 2014.

Internet references

1. http://suzycohen.com/articles/methylation-problems/
2. http://www.webmd.com/vitamins-supplements/ingredientmono-957-RIBOFLAVIN%20(VITAMIN%20B2).aspx?activeIngredientId=957&activeIngredientName=RIBOFLAVIN+(VITAMIN+B2)
3. https://en.wikipedia.org/wiki/Pyridoxal_phosphate
4. http://www.health.harvard.edu/blog/vitamin-b12-deficiency-can-be-sneaky-harmful-201301105780
5. https://en.wikipedia.org/wiki/Spina_bifida
6. https://www.organicfacts.net/health-benefits/minerals/health-benefits-of-magnesium.html
7. http://www.webmd.com/vitamins-supplements/ingredientmono-982-ZINC.aspx?activeIngredientId=982&activeIngredientName=ZINC
8. http://www.drlwilson.com/Articles/Insomnia183.htm

Chapter 38:

Skin

Can I apply Aloe Vera gel on my face overnight?

For most people it is probably safe, but as always there are sensitive individuals who can react to Aloe Vera or some of the ingredients: Aloe Vera side effects. What side effects does Aloe Vera have (1)?

I would suggest you get an organic Aloe Vera gel preparation without any of the chemicals mentioned in the link (parabens etc.) and try it on the back of your hand during the day. If you get itchiness and redness of the skin, wash it off right away and do not use the product anymore: you are allergic to the stuff! But because you were awake, you could notice the reaction. Had you applied it to the face and slept through an allergy at night, you may have a more serious reaction for a few days to come, because you did not wash it off early enough.

Most people though will tolerate Aloe Vera gel.

Internet reference

1. http://thealoeverasite.com/aloe-vera-side-effects.php

Chapter 39:

Sleep

What time does it take to fall asleep?

The answer to this is like a rubber band. Usually it takes an adult 10 to 20 minutes to fall asleep. But this would be a person who is not stressed, whose hormones are balanced and where a certain sleep hygiene is in place.
Older people often are melatonin deficient because in older age the pineal gland does not produce as much melatonin. If you give an older person 3 mg of melatonin they often will now also fall asleep normally.
Children have naturally high melatonin in their system; they tend to fall asleep within 5 to 15 minutes.
People with stress have too much cortisol in their system, which competes with the sleeping hormone melatonin. If thyroid hormones are overactive or underactive this results in insomnia as well. A lack of sex hormones (testosterone in males, estrogen and progesterone in females) leads to sleep problems. Once the hormone deficiencies are corrected with bioidentical hormones, a normal sleeping pattern returns.

What you need to know about sleep

There are a couple of facts that everybody should know about sleep, so you work with nature, not against nature.

1. The way our bodies are hardwired, we need 7 to 8 hours of sleep, but we need to fall asleep between 10 PM and 11 PM.

2. The reason for the relative rigid sleeping schedule time wise is that there is the diurnal hormone rhythm that is dictated by the light of the sun (24 hour cycle). Light going into our eyes and melatonin production from our pineal gland is what keeps the internal clock on time. We all know how we derail when we fly east or west. I am more affected when I fly west than east, but the readjustment takes often one or two weeks for a 9-hour time difference.

3. There is interplay between melatonin and cortisol. These two hormones complement each other. When you sleep melatonin governs and resets the hormones to be ready in the morning. This involves an early testosterone peak for the male; cortisol is released to be ready the moment you wake up, because cortisol, which is produced in the adrenal glands, rules during the day giving us energy. Thyroid hormones also give you energy during the day. As I will explain below, human growth hormone also gives you energy and clears your mind.

4. What is not as much known is that human growth hormone (GH) also gives us energy. There is a main growth hormone release (released as a spurt) between midnight and 3 AM when you're deep asleep. The purpose of that is to get you ready with regard to energy for the next day. If you drink alcohol after 5 PM the afternoon before, you will miss that GH spurt at night and have a hangover (lack of energy the following day). At the 23 Annual World Congress on Anti-Aging Medicine on Dec. 13, 2015 in Las Vegas the

endocrinologist, Dr. Thierry Hertoghe from Belgium gave a talk about GH and sleep.

He mentioned that even one drink the evening before you go to sleep will cancel 75% of the GH spurt causing a lack of energy the following day. When you have alcoholic drinks evening after evening as many people do, you interfere with your deepest sleep (you create a fitful sleep) and you develop GH deficiency, which can be measured in blood and urine. This leads to premature wrinkles, musculoskeletal problems, muscle weakness and dementia. Many aged people in their 80's are not objectively aged, they are growth hormone deficient and could be treated, if confirmed by tests.

5. As we age, we produce less melatonin and less growth hormone. All of these hormone levels can be determined. If they are low they should be replaced with small amounts of the missing hormone (this includes thyroid hormones, sex hormones and DHEA, another energy hormone). This is part of anti-aging medicine. Naturopaths are well versed in this type of approach as well. Whatever you do, don't take sleeping pills, because it only treats you symptomatically, but ultimately make your sleeping problem worse.

What happens when you go to bed late every night?

1. Your body has the built-in diurnal rhythm, which is regulated by the daytime hormone cortisol, which governs your stress responses and the nighttime hormone melatonin, which is produced by the pineal gland. People lose melatonin beyond the age of 10 or 20. Particularly people above the age of 40 or 50, produce very little melatonin in their pineal gland. There are huge variations depending on how much stress there is in your life. The

more high-strung a person is, the more stress there is in his or her life the more difficult it will be to fall asleep and to sleep through.

2. On top of that biological fact there is the area of good habits or bad habits. Some people have no problem disciplining themselves to go to sleep between 10 PM and 11 PM, which seems to be the window of opportunity to catch a good night's sleep. Others are so used to do their late night activities (reading, watching TV, being online, going to the pub etc.) that they finally drop into bed at 1 or 2 AM. People need 7 to 8 hours of good sleep; even celebrities need to get that much sleep. When you go to bed only at 1 AM or 2 AM, it is difficult to get enough sleep.

3. You are asking what the effects are of going to bed late every night. Others have already answered this, so I will not repeat it. But it is true that you can suffer multiple health problems as all the other hormones depend on the resetting during your deepest sleep between 2 AM and 4 AM triggered by the nighttime melatonin response. Even your telomeres, the caps of chromosomes in every cell get shortened from too much stress and too little sleep. Shortened telomeres mean a shortened life span.

4. Here is the solution of what to do: because we mostly have a lack of melatonin, the first step is to take 3mg to 5mg of melatonin at bedtime. But it should be taken during the window of opportunity as mentioned above: between 10 PM and 11 PM. It takes 20 to 30 minutes for melatonin to take effect. If you do not fall asleep within that time frame you are likely thinking too much. If that is the case, I would recommend to take 1 or 2 capsules of valerian root (500 mg strength) from the health food store. This combined with the melatonin should help in more than 80%-90% of insomnia cases. If you cannot sleep, see your physician. You may have to have sleep studies done or you may have problems of the thyroid (hypo- or hyperthyroidism), which

may need to be checked. Other medical problems including depression have to be checked out as well. Melatonin and valerian are safe. Other sleeping pills have multiple side effects including memory problems.

Having said that valerian can have mild side effects like a dry mouth, thinking problems etc. as indicated here (1).

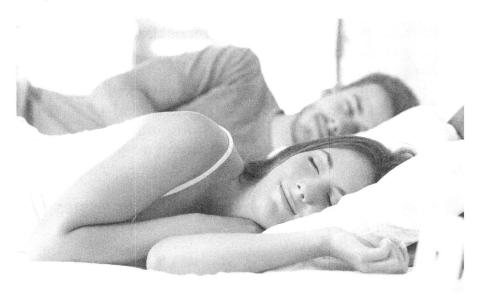

Internet reference

1. https://www.drugs.com/mtm/valerian-root.html

Is going to bed at 5 AM and waking up at 1 PM unhealthy?

When you went to bed at 5 AM, you have disrupted your diurnal hormonal rhythm. This means you missed the human growth hormone peak between midnight and 3 AM, so you won't have the energy you need for the following day despite your 8 hours sleep. You also have not built up the optimal amount of adrenal gland hormones that depend on normal melatonin action during your sleep. But you also need cortisol to give you energy throughout the day. Your hormones are interdependent; they work like clockwork when you go to bed between 10 PM and 11 PM. But when you mess with this internal rhythm, it starts affecting your health (telomere shortening, life expectancy reduced). If you pay attention to your diurnal hormone rhythm it is like an extra asset you have.

As a result, my answer to your question is: yes, it is unhealthy to go to bed at 5 AM and wake up at 1 PM. There is more info about the diurnal hormone rhythm in the question above: "What happens when you go to bed late every night?"

Will a drug ever be developed that eliminates the need for sleep?

1. We will never reach that point where a drug would eliminate the need for sleep. For one thing, drugs always have side effects, whereas hormones don't have side effects when they are balanced.

2. This question has been created by a desire to make your life more efficient and for some reason seems to go around on the Internet.

3. Here is why this is not possible: We need 7 to 8 hours of sleep every night to reset our internal clock, also known as diurnal hormonal rhythm or circadian rhythm. Without that your brain hormones won't work, your body hormones would be disbalanced. You could not function, because your body and brain cells would not function. So, why fight yourself, when this is impossible? You are wasting your time.

Here is more info about sleep: See the answer to the question: "What happens when you go to bed late every night?" above.

Could genetic engineering help humans one day to only need 1 or 2 hours of sleep daily?

This question is another modification of wanting to reduce the amount of sleep people need to restore overnight. The diurnal hormone rhythm dictates that we sleep 7 to 8 hours at night and that sleep is started between 10 PM and 11 PM.

I think it is unlikely that genetic engineering will change the amount of sleep humans need to regenerate. I realize that giraffes and elephants need less sleep than humans, but if you were able to insert the gene for less sleep from an elephant or a giraffe into humans, our hormone requirements and our need for organ rejuvenation would not have changed. You may have succeeded to make us finally sleep less, but you would be burnt out at the age of 40 and die of organ failure. It is at this point in time that scientists will admit that they made a mistake.

Read the answer to the question above: "What you need to know about sleep".

How much would the average person gain from one hour of extra sleep?

Here is how much sleep the average American gets (1).

According to Gallup poll 14% of people get 5 hours sleep or less and 26% of people get 6 hours or less sleep per night (2). That means that 40% of Americans are at risk of getting into health problems because of a lack of sleep.

Your goal should be to sleep at least 7 to 8 hours per night. And the sleep should start between 10 PM and 11 PM. The reason for this is that we are hard-wired with our circadian hormone rhythm to do so.

The circadian hormone rhythm: Here is a brief run-down what that circadian hormone rhythm is. Our nights are ruled by melatonin, the key hormone from the pineal gland that rules like a king over night. It makes sure that we get sleepy when it gets dark and helps us to get the deeper sleep stages later during our sleep. While we sleep between midnight and 3AM, we get a growth hormone (GH) spurt that gives us energy the following day. If you had one alcoholic drink between 5 PM and midnight 75% of the GH is missing as alcohol inhibits the pineal gland to release that GH spurt. If you do that too often, you age faster. In the morning when you open your eyes, light stimulates your retina and this functions like a switch in activating melatonin. At the same time cortisol, the natural counterpart to melatonin, that had time to be built up in your adrenal glands while you slept will be the ruler during the day. So, between melatonin, cortisol and the light from the sun (or artificial light) we regulate our circadian rhythm. If we do not fall asleep between 10 and 11 PM and do not sleep 7 to 8 hours per night, our hormones do not recover optimally overnight. Apart from cortisol and GH the other hormones that give us energy during the day are thyroid hormones, DHEA from the adrenal glands, and our sex hormones (testosterone in males, estrogen and progesterone in females).

Your question answered: You wanted to know how much the average person would benefit from 1 hour extra sleep. 60% of the average Americans get enough sleep. They would benefit from cutting out sugar and engage in regular exercising, but they don't need extra sleep. It is the 40% of people who get less than 7 to 8 hours of sleep who would benefit from the extra hour of sleep (or the group sleeping 5 hours or less perhaps 2 hours extra sleep). What would this do? It would give them the proper GH spurt between midnight and 3AM, would give them enough cortisol and DHEA from the adrenal glands, and add thyroid hormones, and our sex hormones (testosterone in males, estrogen and progesterone in females). In short, this is all required for a full day of energy and protection of our immune system. It will only happen after a full night's restorative sleep!

Here is what you can do, if you are not getting enough sleep, because you have problems falling asleep: Read point 4 of the answer to this question above:

"What happens when you go to bed late every night?"

Internet references

1. https://cbschicago.files.wordpress.com/2014/06/average-sleep-by-age.png
2. http://www.gallup.com/poll/166553/less-recommended-amount-sleep.aspx

What are the nuts and bolts about sleeping?

We need 7 to 8 hours of sleep per night. Sleep research has shown that the best time to fall asleep is between 10 PM and 11 PM. This way your hormones will be reset overnight automatically (diurnal hormone rhythm). Too much stress hormone (cortisol) counters the production of melatonin, the sleep hormone. When people get older, melatonin is not produced as well, but melatonin supplementation will correct this, re-establishing the balance between cortisol and melatonin (see below).

2. People live very busy lives and often push the envelope by staying up late at night. This interferes with your growth hormone release that happens when you

are deep asleep between midnight and 3AM. If you miss this growth hormone spurt, you will have a hangover the following day and a lack of energy all day. If you ignore this and go until the early morning hours again the following day, you start interrupting your normal sleep cycle, get a fitful sleep and wake up several times during the night finding it difficult to fall asleep again.

3. Other hormone deficits also affect your sleeping pattern: a lack of testosterone in males and a lack of estrogen/progesterone in females is what cause sleep disturbances in menopause (in women) and andropause (in men). Low thyroid levels also cause insomnia, which is normalized when thyroid supplementation is given (T3 and T4 mixed). Discuss that with your physician who can order appropriate tests.

Conclusion

We need to be aware how important a proper hormone balance is when it comes to a healthy sleep pattern. Thyroid hormones and the sex hormones are easy to measure. Bioidentical hormone replacement is needed, if one of the hormones is low. Growth hormone is a bit more difficult to assess, but IGF-1 levels give a first indication what your growth hormone levels are doing. The newest test is a 24-hour urine collection looking for growth hormone metabolites. If this is low, daily replacement of growth hormone using a pen similar to insulin injections in diabetics can be given using pure human growth hormone.

Melatonin deficiency in older age is replaced the way I summarized it here: Read point 4 of the answer to this question above:

"What happens when you go to bed late every night?"

I sleep from midnight until 7:30AM, but I am extremely groggy in the morning. Why?

The reason you are groggy in the morning is because you timed your sleep such that you are missing the human growth hormone (HGH) spurt between midnight and 3 AM. Your diurnal hormone rhythm is tightly controlled and releases the HGH spurt only during deep sleep, which takes two to three hours after initiating sleep. If you would go to bed between 10 PM and 11 PM every night, you would gradually correct this problem and you would wake up after 7 to 8 hours of sleep feeling fresh and regenerated. The HGH spike is necessary to give you the energy boost you want for the next day. You are depriving yourself of it every night.

Read a more comprehensive answer of what I summarized above under the question above: "What happens when you go to bed late every night?"

I have to work night shifts (9 PM to 6:30 AM). How will this affect my health?

I realize that you cannot change this or you may lose your job. I would like to be optimistic, but yes, there are health consequences because you are going against what your brain is hardwired for: sleep at night and be awake during the day.

Your body does not care what you want to do; it rewards you, if you sleep 7 to 8 hours during the night and it will penalize you severely, if you turn it upside down. The reason is the diurnal hormone rhythm that we all have built in. Sleep is regulated by melatonin during the night, which is released by the pineal gland located at the base of the skull. Daytime wakefulness is regulated by the stress hormone cortisol from the adrenal glands. These two hormones inhibit each other, cortisol inhibits melatonin and melatonin inhibits cortisol. All the other hormones are also regulated according to the diurnal rhythm: testosterone is highest in the morning, human growth hormone is highest between midnight and 3 AM etc.

There are examples of what happens when you do shift work for several years:

1. A Swedish study found that white-collar shift workers had a 2.6-fold higher mortality over a control group of daytime white-collar workers: Shift work and mortality (1).
2. A study compared night workers in the age group of 45 to 54 with daytime workers and found a 1.47-fold higher mortality rate in the night shift workers: Shift Workers' Mortality Scrutinized (2).

Shift workers do exactly what you are suggesting: they work at night and they sleep during the day. Yes, it can be done, but it is against the physiology of your body as I explained above. Remember that melatonin does not only regulate your sleep, it also is one of the main stimulant hormone of the immune system.

I like to add to this that if you are below 40 years of age, you get away with night shift work for a period of time. I would do it only as long as you really have to do it, because you are slowly shortening your telomeres (the end caps of chromosomes in all of your cells) as the years go by. So, plan ahead and ask yourself what you want to do in 5 years or 10 years from now. I hope it is not nightshift then. One of the peculiar things is that some people have no problems working at nights and sleeping during the day and others have great problems. Ultimately you should listen to your body and observe how you are. Can you tolerate it or not? If you cannot tolerate it, discuss this with your employer. You may be surprised that he/she wants to keep you on and will give you day shift work, because you are a valuable worker.

Conclusion

If you manipulate your diurnal hormone rhythm by staying awake during the night and sleeping during the day, you pay the price by an increased risk of mortality (which means increased risk of death). I think it is not worth it.

Internet references

1. https://www.ncbi.nlm.nih.gov/pubmed/15646250
2. http://www.tandfonline.com/doi/abs/10.1081/CBI-200035942

Why do we have to sleep 7-8 hours a night, why not just 4 hours?

The reason we need 7 to 8 hours of sleep at night is the diurnal hormone rhythm. Sleep is there to regenerate your body. Part of this is a resetting of your hormone system while you sleep. Part of this is the human growth hormone that is only released between midnight and 3 AM during your deepest sleep (REM sleep). HGH gives you the energy for the following day together with cortisol. Your sex hormones are regenerated early in the morning before you wake up. Cortisol is built up in your adrenal glands all night long while melatonin is high in your blood system (melatonin and cortisol are opposing each other: when cortisol is high in the blood, melatonin is low and vice versa).

In addition your brain needs downtime as well to regenerate all of the brain hormones while you sleep.

Best go to sleep between 10 PM and 11 PM and sleep for 7 to 8 hours every night!

More info: read the chapter above: What are the nuts and bolts about sleeping?

Publications of medical questions and answers in popular magazines.

Forbes.com: June 20, 2017

What Happens To Your Body If You Get Fewer Than Six Hours Of Sleep Every Night?

Answer by Ray Schilling, M.D., author of "Healing Gone Wrong, Healing Done Right".

Will getting less than six hours of sleep every night for many consecutive years affect a person? These studies say yes!

Sleep deprivation in nursing homes

A publication has zeroed in on what happens in the frail elderly who live in nursing homes (1).
Here is what sleep researchers have found:

- Older people need 7 to 8 hours of sleep per night, not less as previously thought.
- Let people sleep at night, and give them undisturbed sleep. The practice of waking them up every 2 hours is unnecessary and undermines a restful sleep with normal amounts of REM sleep.
- The color of light matters: Blue/purple light coming from TVs, iPod's, laptops or cell phones stimulates serotonin production that wakes you up. In contrast to this, orange/red light stimulates melatonin production that facilitates sleep. A nursing home owner, Guildermann said: "We have made it darker at night, and what light they do have is orange/amber/red light, and we are having phenomenal results".

- Sleep, exercise and nutrition are the biggest components of health.

Night workers

- One of the news stories in 2016 was about health risks of night shifts (2). The Bureau of Labor Statistics reported in 2000 that 15 million workers (16.8 % of the working population) were doing alternative shifts (night shift work mixed with daytime shifts). In 2016 they reported 14.8% were working alternate shifts. Among blacks, Asians and Latino Americans the percentage of working alternative shifts was higher, namely 20.8%, 15.7% and 16%, respectively.
- Shift work is more common in certain industries, such as protective services like the police force, food services, health services and transportation.
- Your body rewards you when you sleep 7 to 8 hours during the night, but it will penalize you severely, if you turn it upside down. The reason is because of the diurnal hormone rhythm that we all have built in. Sleep is regulated by melatonin during the night, which is released by the pineal gland (on the base of the skull). Daytime wakefulness is regulated by the stress hormone cortisol from the adrenal glands. These two hormones inhibit each other, cortisol inhibits melatonin and melatonin inhibits cortisol. All the other hormones are also regulated according to the diurnal rhythm: testosterone, for instance is highest in the morning, human growth hormone is highest between midnight and 3 AM.
- There are examples of what happens when you do shift work for several years:
A) A Swedish study found that white-collar shift workers

had a 260% higher mortality compared to a control group of daytime white collar workers (3).

B) A study compared night workers in the age group of 45 to 54 with daytime workers and found a 147% higher mortality rate in the night shift workers (4).

Shift workers work at night and sleep during the day. This can be done, but it is against the physiology of your body, as I explained above. Remember that melatonin does not only regulate your sleep, it also is one of the main stimulant hormones of the immune system. If you manipulate your diurnal hormone rhythm by staying awake during the night and sleeping during the day, you pay the price by an increased risk of mortality (increased risk of death). This is not worth it!

Telomere length and sleep deficit.

- It is true that you can suffer multiple health problems with insufficient sleep, as all of your hormones depend on the resetting during your deepest sleep between 2AM and 4AM triggered by the nighttime melatonin response. Even your telomeres, the caps of chromosomes in every cell get shortened from too much stress and too little sleep (5).
- Shortened telomeres mean a shortened life span. The reason for this is that people with shortened telomeres develop heart attacks, strokes and cancer. How do we avoid this risk? Develop healthy sleep habits. It is best to start going to sleep between 10 PM and 11 PM and sleep for 7 to 8 hours.

Conclusion

It appears that there are health consequences for only sleeping 6 hours every night instead of 7 to 8 hours.

More info here (6).

Internet references

1. http://www.nextavenue.org/know-poor-sleep-older-adults/
2. https://www.medicalnewstoday.com/articles/288310.php
3. http://www.tandfonline.com/doi/abs/10.1081/CBI-200035942
4. http://www.tandfonline.com/doi/abs/10.1081/CBI-200035942
5. http://journals.plos.org/plosone/article?id=10.1371%2Fjournal.pone.0047292
6. http://www.askdrray.com/results-of-insomnia-studies/

I don't sleep well, I am unhappy and I lost my zest for life. What should I do?

1. I would suggest you discuss this with your doctor. You need professional help for your emotional problems. It needs to be discussed through. The best is to find a therapist who practices cognitive/behavioral therapy. Your doctor can also decide whether or not you ill need in addition anti-depressant medicine for a period of time.
2. If you have problems sleeping, melatonin is useful as is the herb valerian. I have described this under point 4 of this link: What happens when you go to bed late every night?
3. Be patient. It may take several weeks before you will feel better. You need regular sleep and you need a better mood. Both can be achieved with what I recommended.

If I sleep for 6 hours, am I getting enough sleep?

No, 6 hours of sleep is not enough. You may think it is enough, but your diurnal hormone rhythm will disagree. You need to go to bed between 10 PM and 11 PM and sleep for about 7 to 8 hours to keep your hormones in balance. If you work with your hormones, you will feel energy and feel good about yourself. More info about sleep:
"What are the nuts and bolts about sleeping?"

Chapter 40:

Sugar

Will I be OK living without sugar?

If you want to live longer, get rid of all sugar in your diet and also keep the consumption of starchy foods extremely low. Stick to low-glycemic foods as these have been shown to be the healthiest carbs. Low carb foods will lower your LDL cholesterol and your triglycerides. This puts you into a much lower risk category to get a heart attack or a stroke.

It also makes you lose some weight. (I had to have my clothes taken in several times when my wife and I embarked on this low-glycemic diet in 2001).

How you would go shopping for low glycemic food is summarized in this section above under "diets": I want to get rid of sugar in my diet. How can I do this long-term?

Effects of sugar on our health

1. Sugar overconsumption is the problem. A 2015 study showed that worldwide 184,000 deaths per year are attributable to sugar-sweetened beverage consumption; among those there are 133,000 deaths from diabetes, 45,000 deaths from cardiovascular disease and 6,450 deaths

from cancers. Estimated Global, Regional, and National Disease Burdens Related to Sugar-Sweetened Beverage Consumption in 2010 (1). Those people who developed disabilities from strokes, heart attacks, osteoporosis and severe arthritis measured 8.5 million disability-adjusted life years throughout the world and were related to sugar-sweetened beverages. 4.5% of these were from diabetes that was related to sugar-sweetened beverages. Even cancer can be caused from sugar overconsumption: Sugar As A Cause Of Cancer (2).

2. Advanced glycation end products (AGEs) form when food is cooked at high temperatures. Sugar molecules react with proteins cross-linking them and changing how they function. It prevents proteins from doing their job. Glycation also causes inflammation, which damages mitochondria, the power packages inside cells that provide the body with energy. Overall AGEs lead to premature aging, which comes from the toxic protein reactions. Advanced glycation end products accumulate as glycated proteins in the tissues of the body. This leads to mitochondrial dysfunction. More info here (3). The bottom line is that mitochondrial loss in body cells leads to shorter life expectancy due to more heart attacks, strokes, diabetes and Alzheimer's.

3. Sugar consumption has skyrocketed over the past 100 years. An entirely new recommendation of the FDA is that sugar should be reduced in anybody's diet. The FDA explains that sugar is contained in too many processed foods, is added in drinks like coffee, fruit juices, food items like muffins and cakes. In the past decades it has become clear that it is sugar that is much more the culprit than fat, when it comes to hardening of arteries. Sugar gets metabolized in the liver, triglycerides and LDL cholesterol are increased, and this gets deposited into arteries and fatty tissue. The sugar industry has funded fake research papers for years to confuse the consumer. In this context

it makes sense that the FDA now recommends a reduction of sugar intake.

4. The American Heart Association has recently recommended the following limits for sugar consumption:
- For men: a daily dose of 9 teaspoons of sugar from all foods.
- For women: a daily dose of 6 teaspoons of sugar from all foods.

Conclusion

We are in the middle of an obesity wave caused by sugar overconsumption. We need to cut out the low fat/high carb diet, which was erroneously recommended in the 1980's and 1990's. Replace it with a Mediterranean diet (low carb, medium healthy fat diet), which has been found to be anti-inflammatory. Humans have over consumed sugar in form of processed foods and added sugar products for the last 100 years. We need to limit our added sugar intake to the recommendations mentioned above by the American Heart Association. This will lower heart attacks, diabetes, obesity, strokes, Alzheimer's disease and many cancers. As a result your life expectancy will be 10 to 20 years longer without any of these major diseases.

Internet references

1. https://www.ncbi.nlm.nih.gov/pubmed/26124185
2. http://www.askdrray.com/sugar-as-a-cause-of-cancer/
3. http://www.askdrray.com/advanced-glycation-end-products-ages/
4. http://www.heart.org/HEARTORG/HealthyLiving/HealthyEating/Nutrition/Added-Sugars_UCM_305858_Article.jsp#.WiTdWrT80Uv

If I cut out sugar, what will happen?

1. If you stop eating sugar, you will lose a few pounds. You will initially miss the sugar-fix, but you can overcome that within 1 to 2 weeks by eating protein and fat containing snacks. Snacks with yogurt, ricotta cheese, cheese slices and vegetables will help to overcome the sugar craving. Nuts or almonds are also a good snack.

2. Your energy will increase. Your mood will stabilize, and you will be less anxious. There is really nothing to fear. I know from the medical literature that the risk for heart attacks and strokes goes down, because the triglyceride and LDL cholesterol levels normalize.

3. I got rid of sugar in my diet in 2001. I lost 50 pounds in 3 months. And I kept it down. I am still off sugar and starchy foods. I use stevia powder, if I need a sweet taste. This is metabolically neutral compared to sugar, which causes an insulin reaction.

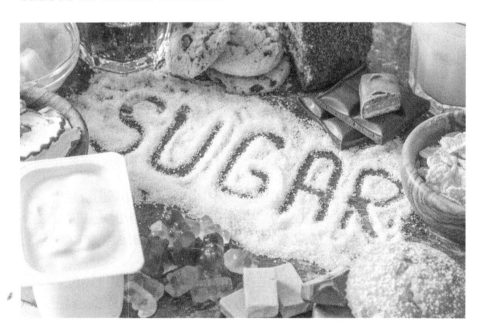

Chapter 41:

Vaccinations

Is there a connection between vaccinations and autism?

10 to 15 years ago this was a hypothesis. But it has been proven to be wrong.
1. In the meantime, due to mounting pressure from the public, most vaccines no longer contain thimerosal, the mercury preservative compound. Yet the autism rate continues to climb. This would imply that there is another mechanism that causes autism.
2. There have been large trials that showed that there is no correlation between the amount of vaccinations a child gets and autism (1).
3. This leaves the question of what causes autism? The strongest factor seems genetic factors, but there could be epigenetic factors (environmental modifications of genetic traits) that play a role (2).Research is still ongoing. A defect in metal processing metabolism has been identified to be a cause in some with autism (3).
4. Despite all of the research there is no clear-cut answer to what causes autism and what would be an effective treatment. Many children were treated with intravenous

chelation and they improved drastically. This points to the importance of removing heavy metals from the body, because that is what chelation therapy does.

Internet references

1. https://www.cdc.gov/vaccinesafety/concerns/autism.html
2. https://en.wikipedia.org/wiki/Causes_of_autism
3. http://www.healing-arts.org/children/metal-metabolism.htm

Chapter 42:

Vitamins and Supplements

Are taking vitamins and supplements healthy or are they harmful?

Vitamin and supplements have shown to extend telomeres and over a lifetime may add about 5 years to your life expectancy. Here is an overview of the more important vitamins and supplements with an explanation of how they work.

Vitamins and supplements needed for heart attack and stroke prevention

1. Vitamin K2 has emerged in several studies as an important vitamin that removes calcium from the vascular compartment and transports it into the bones where it is stored. Osteoporosis prevention is closely linked to heart attack and stroke prevention, which in my opinion is not widely known. Another study from 2013 was using a much larger patient base of 36,282 postmenopausal women of the Women's Health initiative in the US who were followed up for 7 years. Initially there was some confusion as to how compliant the patients were in taking the required

1000 mg of calcium carbonate and 400 IU of vitamin D3. The supplement compliant group, when compared 7 years into the trial, had 35% to 38% less fractures of the hip than the placebo group. This supplementation did not cause kidney stones in the study group, as is often cited by some physicians as the reason why they do not want to recommend supplementing with vitamin D3 and calcium. In other words, all the stories about these kidney stone concerns you have so often read in the media are not true.

2. The second vitamin needed is vitamin D3 in doses of 4000 IU to 5000 IU per day. This helps to absorb calcium in the gut, but also helps to transport it into the bones away from the arteries. Apart from these vitamins and supplements regular exercise is needed to condition heart and lungs. The overall effect is that osteoporosis, heart attacks and strokes are prevented. Keep in mind that sugar needs to be avoided as well to prevent oxidation of LDL cholesterol.

3. PQQ and Co-Q-10 are also needed for heart attack and stroke prevention (see below). These two supplements strengthen the mitochondria, the tiny power packages within the heart muscle cells and the brain cells. The better the support, the more resilient the heart and the brain are to the changes when a person is aging. The heart and the brain are particularly rich in mitochondria.

4. Vitamin D3, alpha-lipoic acid and resveratrol are also needed for prevention of heart attacks and strokes, because of the anti-inflammatory action (see below).

5. Magnesium and green leaf tea extract have been proven to be beneficial in terms of preventing heart attacks.

6. Hawthorn is an herb that has been found useful for prevention of heart disease and treatment of mild heart failure (1). It is available as a supplement in capsules at health food stores.

Mitochondrial function needs to be improved

If we want to have energy when we age, we need to take care of our mitochondria. This is where the biochemical processes take place that produce energy for us.

There are several steps and supplements that will help us preserve mitochondria:

1. Mitochondrial aging is slowed down by ubiquinol (=Co-Q-10). Co-Q-10 repairs DNA damage to your mitochondria.

2. Another supplement, PQQ (=Pyrroloquinoline quinone) stimulates your healthy mitochondria to multiply. Between the two supplements you will have more energy as optimal mitochondrial function is ensured.

3. There are simple lifestyle changes you can make: eat less calories as this will stimulate the genes, which in turn stimulates your cell metabolism including the mitochondria.

4. Resveratrol, the supplement from red grape skin, can also stimulate your mitochondria metabolism. Build regular exercise into your life style, as this will also stimulate your mitochondria to multiply similar to the effects of PQQ.

5. Alpha-lipoic acid is an anti-oxidant that counters the slowdown of mitochondrial metabolism.

Anti-inflammatory vitamins and supplements

Since the mid 1990's it is known by the medical profession that inflammation plays an important role in the development of heart attacks, strokes, inflammatory bowel diseases like Crohn's disease and ulcerative colitis, Alzheimer's disease, diabetes mellitus, arthritis (both rheumatoid arthritis and osteoarthritis), multiple sclerosis, just to name a few. Here is a list of vitamins and supplements that counter inflammation:

1. Vitamin D3 is an anti-inflammatory helping to prevent heart disease and cancer (2).
2. Alpha-lipoic acid: This anti-inflammatory is both water and oil soluble (3). It is an antioxidant protecting from cardiovascular disease, diabetes, and may reduce the size of a stroke.
3. Bioflavonoids are found in fruit and vegetables (4). One of the most potent ones is resveratrol. Resveratrol prevents oxidation of LDL cholesterol, which prevents heart attacks (5). It also prevents Alzheimer's disease and helps prevent insulin resistance.
4. Garlic: This herb has anti-inflammatory effects, stimulates the immune system and lowers blood pressure moderately (6). It is used as an adjunct in treating high blood pressure, prevents heart disease and various cancers. It helps to reduce inflammation with osteoarthritis.
5. Ginger root extract: Ginger root is an anti-inflammatory, but also has anti-nausea effects and is useful for seasickness, morning sickness and side-effects from chemotherapy (7). Arthritis is also helped by it.
6. Ginseng is a popular herbal medicine; it has anti-inflammatory effects and improves immune function (8). Often people take it during the cold and flu season.
7. Green tea extract is anti-inflammatory and has anti-oxidant effects (9). It is used for cancer prevention, stomach upsets, and diarrhea. It also helps in patients with Crohn's disease and helps prevent heart disease.
8. Melatonin is a natural hormone produced in the pineal gland (10). It is a powerful anti-oxidant and anti-inflammatory. It also helps you to sleep. In higher doses it is used as anti-cancer medicine as it stimulates the immune system.
9. Rutin is a bioflavonoid that is used to strengthen blood vessels, helps in stroke prevention and helps with osteoarthritis (11).

10. Selenium is a trace element and an important antioxidant and anti-inflammatory (12). It stimulates the immune system, helps in prevention of cancer, and converts T4 thyroid hormone into the more active T3 thyroid hormone.

11. Cod liver oil (omega-3) and krill oil are both omega-3 fatty acids (13). Krill oil contains more DHA, while fish oil derived omega-3 fatty acids contains more omega-3. Both krill oil and fish oil are needed as supplements to prevent arthritis, strokes, heart attacks, osteoporosis, diabetes, dementia, Alzheimer's and inflammation.

12. Coenzyme Q10 has antioxidant properties, but also anti-inflammatory properties and helps to prevent cancer and heart disease (14).

13. Flax seed: Ground flax seed has anti-inflammatory omega-3 in it, cancer-protective lignans, blood pressure lowering properties and mild blood thinning activity (15). Flax seed has a rather tough shell. With a cheap coffee grinder you can easily grind your flax seed. In a few seconds it is ground. It is important to wipe out the grinder after use with a damp cloth to prevent future rancidity of leftover ground flax seed. It can be incorporated into breakfast smoothies or sprinkled on oatmeal or muesli. Using flaxseed in baked or cooked food cancels the benefits. Consume it freshly ground!

Some people are born with enzymatic defects in the methylation pathways (16). They are more prone to diverse diseases like autism, depression, anxiety, schizophrenia, adrenal dysfunction, addiction, cancer, allergies, immune weakness, diabetes etc.

Here is a list of the methylation pathway vitamins and trace elements important for those who are born into families where mental illness or diabetes is frequent, as they are the ones who often have methylation defects. But many of those defects can be corrected (Ref.1).

1. Vitamin B2/riboflavin: Riboflavin is used for neonatal jaundice as part of phototherapy. Some adult patients experience relief from migraines (17).

2. Vitamin B6/pyridoxine: Pyridoxal phosphateis a co-factor of many enzymatic reactions in amino acid, glucose and lipid metabolism (18).

3. Vitamin B12/methylcobalamin: Vitamin B12 is essential for your nerve function, bone marrow function, or severe anemia follows (19). It gives you energy, but it is not a cure all. Sometimes in older patients absorption is a problem, but B12 injections every couple of months can easily overcome this.

4. Folate (from food or folic acid): Research about neural tube defects (spina bifida) in the baby of a folate deficient mother led to the discovery of folic acid (20). Heavy smokers and drinkers can get folate deficient. Folate is needed in DNA synthesis.

5. Magnesium is involved in more than 300 biochemical reactions within the body. It helps with asthma, bone heath, muscle pain and prevents heart attacks (21). In psychiatric disease like anxiety and agitation it is an adjunct to treatment. Magnesium is a co-factor for many enzymes reactions.

6. Zinc: Because zinc is an essential trace element, it is involved in many organ systems, and zinc is used for many health problems (22). People may have heard that zinc is an important supplement in male infertility and erectile dysfunction. But it is also needed as a supplement in diabetes, high blood pressure, psoriasis, macular degeneration and night blindness. Zinc is a natural opponent of copper meaning that when zinc is low, copper levels in the blood are often high. This constellation can cause insomnia (23).

What makes a vitamin or supplement an anti-aging product?

If a vitamin or supplement fits into one of these following classes, it helps slow down aging and for this reason would be considered an anti-aging product:

1. Antioxidants (fight oxidant stress): a typical representative would be vitamin C, which prevents oxidative damage of our DNA. Others are B vitamins (B1, B3, B6, B12 and folate), acetyl-L-carnitine, alpha-lipoic acid, bioflavonoid, garlic, ginger root extract, Gingko biloba, ginseng, green tea extract, L-glutathione, magnesium, manganese, melatonin, N-acetyl cysteine, potassium, rutin, selenium, vitamin E, and coenzyme Q10. We have discussed them above.

2. Anti-inflammatory action (fighting inflammation): vitamin D3 comes to mind, which suppresses inflammation in nerves (MS) or in blood vessels preventing heart disease. Others are alpha-lipoic acid, bioflavonoid, garlic, ginger root extract, ginseng, green tea extract, melatonin, rutin, selenium, cod liver oil (omega-3), coenzyme Q10, and ground flax seed.

3. Preserving mitochondrial function: B-vitamins and coenzyme Q10 are examples that do this. Mitochondria are important to provide energy in the body. Others are acetyl-L-carnitine, alpha-lipoic acid, ginger root extract, ginseng and selenium.

4. There are vitamins and supplements that will prevent insulin resistance. This is pretty important, as diabetes, where insulin resistance is present, will shorten life expectancy. Ginseng, green tea extract and magnesium are examples of supplements that prolong life through countering insulin resistance. Others that do this are B vitamins (B1, B3, B6, B12 and folate), vitamin D, alpha-

lipoic acid, beta-carotene, chromium picolinate, garlic, ginger root extract, manganese, potassium, and selenium.

5. Other supplements are prolonging life by providing membrane integrity: beta-carotene, garlic and selenium belong into this group. Others are ginger root extract, ginseng, cod liver oil (omega-3), and ground flax seed.

6. Partial methylation defects can be cured with B vitamins explained earlier and this has been shown to help improve some mental disorders significantly, improve life quality, prevent suicides and prolong life.

Many vitamins and supplements have not only an action in one of those categories, but in two or more. B1, B3, B6, B12 and folate belong into category 1, 3, 4 and 6, so there is a huge overlap, and this is what anti-aging physicians consider an advantage. Often conventional physicians shake their heads and say that the overlapping actions would prove that they are worthless. However, as time went on conventional physicians have started to adopt more and more the anti-aging concept, mostly because science is proving in large trials from the Karolinska Institute in Sweden (24), from various Chinese universities (25), from American universities like Loyola University (26) and Harvard Medical School (27),Salk Institute (28) and others that the overlapping concept is valid.

If this list sounds intimidatingly long, you can relax! Because of the overlapping effect of vitamins and supplements you may not need to take all of these listed here as long as you have a good overlap (29).

Book reference

Ref. 1: Barry Sears: "The age-free zone". Regan Books, Harper Collins, 2000.
Also see Dr. Sears' website (https://www.drsears.com/).

Internet references

1. https://www.drugs.com/npc/hawthorn.html
2. https://www.ncbi.nlm.nih.gov/books/NBK56061/
3. http://www.natmedtalk.com/showthread.php?t=4923
4. https://www.everydayhealth.com/drugs/bioflavonoids
5. https://www.webmd.com/vitamins-supplements/ingredientmono-307-resveratrol.aspx?activeingredientid=307&activeingredientname=resveratrol
6. https://www.reference.com/health/health-benefits-garlic-31c0f2c7382acfdf?aq=benefit+of+garlic+in+the+body&qo=cdpArticles
7. https://en.wikipedia.org/wiki/Ginger
8. https://www.webmd.com/diet/supplement-guide-ginseng#1
9. https://www.webmd.com/food-recipes/features/health-benefits-of-green-tea#1
10. http://www.doctoroz.com/article/fact-sheet-melatonin
11. https://www.webmd.com/vitamins-supplements/altmodmono-270-RUTIN.aspx?altModalityId=270&altModalityName=RUTIN&source=0
12. https://en.wikipedia.org/wiki/Selenium
13. https://chriskresser.com/the-definitive-fish-oil-buyers-guide/
14. https://en.wikipedia.org/wiki/Coenzyme_Q10
15. https://www.webmd.com/vitamins-supplements/ingredientmono-991-flaxseed.aspx?activeingredientid=991&activeingredientname=flaxseed
16. https://suzycohen.com/articles/snpsmethylation/
17. https://www.webmd.com/vitamins-supplements/altmodmono-957-RIBOFLAVIN.aspx?altModalityId=957&altModalityName=RIBOFLAVIN&source=0
18. https://en.wikipedia.org/wiki/Pyridoxal_phosphate

19. https://www.health.harvard.edu/blog/vitamin-b12-deficiency-can-be-sneaky-harmful-201301105780
20. https://en.wikipedia.org/wiki/Spina_bifida
21. https://www.organicfacts.net/health-benefits/minerals/health-benefits-of-magnesium.html
22. https://www.webmd.com/vitamins-supplements/altmodmono-982-ZINC.aspx?altModalityId=982&altModalityName=ZINC&source=0
23. http://www.drlwilson.com/articles/insomnia183.htm
24. http://ki-su-arc.se/
25. https://academic.oup.com/ajcn/article/89/6/1857/4596854?sid=9aab0e13-b4d2-42ad-b44c-15cffc6771c3
26. https://luc.edu/wellness/services/nutrition/
27. https://www.health.harvard.edu/staying-healthy/supplements-a-scorecard
28. http://nutritionreview.org./2015/07/scientists-discover-on-off-switch-for-controlling-cell-aging/
29. http://www.lifeextension.com/magazine/2012/5/Nutrient-Cocktail-Delays-Aging-Extends-Life-Span/Page-01

The all-important vitamin D

Vitamin D is absorbed in the gut and also is made from ultraviolet light in the skin. The active compound of vitamin D is vitamin D3 (or cholecalciferol). There are vitamin D3 receptors all over the body, which tells you that vitamin D3 is very important. Vitamin D3 is important for the absorption of calcium from the gut. Vitamin D3 is also important for the calcium metabolism within the body. Together with vitamin K2 calcium is mobilized from arteries, is transported into the bones and deposited in bones. This is important for prevention of osteoporosis (1).

Vitamin D3 also stimulates and maintains the immune system. The amount of daily vitamin D3 supplementation is something, which not every health provider agrees with. In the past it was recommended that 400 IU of vitamin D3 would be sufficient. However, these guidelines have undergone an adjustment, as the dosage has been found insufficient to be effective. Generally supplements of vitamin D3 of 5000 IU to 8000 IU are the norm now. But some patients are poor absorbers and they may require 15,000 IU per day. What the patients need in the dosage of vitamin D3 can be easily determined by doing repeat vitamin D blood levels (as 25-hydroxy vitamin D). The goal is to reach a level of vitamin D of 50-80 ng/ml. The optimal level with regard to nmol/L is 80 to 200 (according to Rocky Mountain Analytical, Calgary, AB, Canada).

Internet reference

1. http://www.askdrray.com/calcium-vitamin-d3-and-vitamin-k2-needed-for-bone-health/

Why does turmeric fight cancer?

At this point in time curcumin, which is the most powerful antioxidant of turmeric has absorption problems and problems of persistently showing anti-cancer activities. Below I have reviewed the literature about curcumin.

Introduction

Many clinicians give their attention to curcumin and cancer. It may not be used as a primary treatment, but may be added as an adjunct to other cancer treatments. Curcumin is the effective ingredient of the old Indian spice, turmeric. The question is how effective curcumin is against cancer? Is it safe to use? What is the evidence?

Frequency of cancer

According to the American Cancer Society there will be 1,688,780 new cancer cases diagnosed in 2017 and 600,920 cancer deaths will occur in the US.

Causes of cancer

Cancer can be caused in many different ways. Hidden in the many causes may be the possible solution to new cures.

1. A lack of exercise may contribute to the development of cancer because of a lack of tissue circulation. And exercise will help to support your normal cell metabolism (explained below). Wrong foods may or may not have a contributory role regarding cancer development (a high sugar and starch diet causing insulin response, which changes the metabolism). The Mediterranean diet is an anti-inflammatory diet and has been credited to prevent a lot of cancers (1).

2. Cancer can be caused by chemicals, called carcinogens. But it can also be caused by oncoviruses. It can be genetically caused, that's why it tends to run more often in certain cancer prone families. But Warburg has researched the metabolism of cancer almost 100 years ago, even got the Nobel price for it in 1931, and yet the elusive cancer cure has not materialized yet.

3. Following Warburg's research Watson/Crick detected DNA in our cells. Ever since geneticists were fascinated by it. They also found that a cancer suppressive gene, regulated by the p53 gene could develop mutations and then cancer would occur: the idea of Tumor Suppressor Genes has been the "in" thing for decades. But in the last 5 to 10 years there is a revitalization of the original Warburg idea

that one should concentrate on the metabolic differences between cancer cells and normal cells. This is gradually starting to show some results.

4. Cancer cells are more acidic from lactic acid and burn glucose for energy without requiring oxygen (anaerobic pathway), while normal cells burn glucose in the aerobic pathway in the mitochondria. This difference is important. Cancer cells were found to be more vulnerable to be killed by certain manipulations.

5. Take the example of cryoablation therapy for prostate cancer. The more vulnerable cancer cells are preferentially killed over the normal cells through a local deep freeze method. Another example is phototherapy treatment of cancer that has been used for lung cancer and esophageal cancer (2). This method may be a lot more universally applicable than believed so far. A photosensitized dye is injected and later when normal cells have eliminated the dye, but the defective cancer cells are still containing the dye, a laser beam is used to kill the cancer cells preferentially, absorbing the specific laser wavelength that is specific for the dye.

6. Nobody knows which way cancer research is going. But I think it will be consumer driven: consumers want better cures, and when new methods appear that have better cure rates, these will be pushed forward while less effective methods will become history. I think that Warburg will be revitalized and new therapies will continue to be developed from this as I indicated.

Curcumin and cancer: malignant conversion

There are three development stages for any cancer to develop (3).

This was originally researched with skin cancer, but also confirmed with cervical cancer. It is called the "malignant conversion" that needs to take place before a normal cell has become a cancer cell. There are three stages.

- Initiation
- Promotion
- Progression

This is important to know in the context of curcumin. Basic research has shown that curcumin interferes with all of these stages of tumor development, both in terms of prevention as well as in terms of being curative (4). Here is a link that points out the complex multiple steps of cancer growth that curcumin interferes with (5).

As can be seen from it, curcumin interferes with the initiation of multiple cancers, reduces inflammation, and interferes with angiogenesis and this reduces the amount of metastases that can form. But curcumin further interferes with proliferation of cancer cells, reduces invasion, prevents resistance and improves survival. The underlying molecular and genetic reasons for curcumin's actions are all contained in that link.

Curcumin and cancer: research in tissue culture and animal experiments

When it comes to cancer research, you usually hear about in vitro culture experiments and animal experiments. This type of research is used to establish that there is an anti-cancer effect, that it is reproducible and non-toxic. The September issue of the 2016 Life Extension Magazine reviewed this in detail. It was entitled "How Curcumin Targets Cancer" (6).

Vitamins and Supplements

But as a former clinician I am more interested in seeing cancer patients cured. This has to be verified by clinical trials first. When I looked through Home - PubMed - NCBI (7) for objective evidence of the effects of curcumin in cancer patients, this type of information was more difficult to find. But in the following there are a number of examples that I did find.

Curcumin and cancer: clinical trials

1. Reduction of tumor necrosis factor-alpha

A 2016 meta-analysis of eight randomized studies investigated the effect of curcumin in patients with various inflammatory diseases including cancer (8). They found that curcumin consistently reduced tumor necrosis factor-alpha. In cancer patients this inflammatory substance is responsible for further cancer growth and developments of metastases.

2. Poor bioavailability of curcumin

A study with increasing amounts of curcumin showed poor absorption of curcumin into the blood (9). In this study dosages between 500 mg up to 12,000 mg of curcumin were given per day. 500 mg to 8000 mg of curcumin did not result in any positive serum level of curcumin. Only the higher dosages, 10,000 and 12,000 mg of curcumin were associated with positive curcumin levels in the blood serum. In order to have effects of curcumin, higher amounts have to be taken. Higher amounts of curcumin have been tested for toxicity and were found to be safe and were also fairly well tolerated.

3. Precancerous colonic polyps reduced in number and size

A smaller study consisted of 5 subjects with familial adenomatous polyposis (FAP). This is an autosomal-dominant disorder where hundreds of colorectal adenomas develop in the lining of the colon. From these colorectal cancer can arise. Five patients received 480 mg of curcumin and 20 mg quercetin orally three times per day (10). After 6 months the number of polyps and the size had reduced by 60.4%.

4. Premalignant colonic lesions suppressed by curcumin

44 eligible smoker subjects received a baseline colonoscopy where aberrant crypt foci (ACF) were determined (11). ACI are the very first focal areas in the colon from which colon cancer develops. Smokers are known to have more of these lesions, which was the reason that smoker subjects were used for this trial. The patients received either a supplement of 2000 mg of curcumin or 4000 mg of curcumin for 30 days. These are fairly high doses, but they were used to overcome the poor absorption of curcumin. Colonoscopies were done again after one month of curcumin supplementation. 41 subjects completed the study. In the 4000 mg curcumin group the ACF numbers were reduced significantly by 40%, compared to the 2000 mg group, which showed no reduction. The 4000 mg group showed a 5-fold increase of curcumin blood levels compared to baseline. There was no change in blood levels in the 2000 mg group.

5. Reduction of radiation dermatitis with radiation therapy in breast cancer patients

30 breast cancer patients were divided into an experimental group and a placebo group. All of them had a mastectomy first, which was followed by radiation therapy (12). The experimental group received 6 grams (2 grams three times per day) of curcumin during the time of radiotherapy following mastectomy. The severity of radiation dermatitis following radiotherapy was significantly reduced in the experimental group when compared to the placebo group. In the curcumin group only 28.6% had significant radiation dermatitis versus 87.5% in the placebo group.

6. Chronic multiple myeloma patients

An Australian study involving chronic multiple myeloma patients found that curcumin at 4 Grams per day and even more so at 8 Grams per day stabilized the disease and improved kidney function (13).

7. Descriptive studies

Descriptive studies investigating the effect of various doses of curcumin have been done regarding breast cancer (14), and advanced pancreatic cancer (15). But these clinical trials were all rather small.

8. Chemoprevention of cancer

A phase II trial enrolled 21 patients with end-stage pancreatic cancer (16). The only FDA approved treatments for this are gemcitabine and erlotinib, but this would normally only lead to clinical responses in less than 10% of patients. In this study the investigators used curcumin to enhance the anti-tumor response of either gemcitabine or erlotinib. The study summary stated: "Oral curcumin is well tolerated and, despite its limited absorption, has biological activity in some patients with pancreatic cancer". 2 of the 21 patients had stable disease for more than 18 months; one of the 21 patients had a brief tumor regression of 78%, but then relapsed and died.

9. Chemoprevention of prostate cancer

Chemoprevention of cancer is discussed in this publication (17): There was specific reference made to prevention of prostate cancer and the opinion of the researchers was: "At present, there is no convincing clinical proof or evidence that the cited phytochemicals might be used in an attempt to cure cancer of the prostate".

Conclusion

For years there have been reports to indicate that curcumin was a promising natural supplement that can improve cancer survival. There are poorly founded reports of effects of curcumin on colorectal cancer, pancreas cancer, prostate cancer, breast cancer, ovarian cancer and others. But on closer look the hype seems to come mostly from in vitro studies (tissue culture experiments) or from animal studies. Clinicians, however, demand well-constructed randomized clinical trials with clear research objectives before they can accept a new agent like curcumin to be effective. These clinical trials are missing! Instead there are many in-between trials of questionable quality as listed above.

There have been problems of bioavailability due to poor absorption of curcumin. To a certain extent this could be overcome by pushing the dosage to 6000 to 8000 mg per day. But a significant percentage of people (around 30%) suffered from abdominal cramps and nausea and had to discontinue these high doses of curcumin. Newer curcumin compounds have been developed, but at this point it is not known what the bioequivalent dosage is of these newer curcumin agents in comparison to the original curcumin dosages.

It is quite possible that new trials will one day be performed that may bring better news on survival rates of various cancer patients involving curcumin therapy. But in my opinion right now it is not yet prime time for curcumin!

Internet references

1. https://www.health.harvard.edu/blog/mediterranean-diet-may-prevent-breast-cancer-but-there-are-other-reasons-to-pour-on-the-olive-oil-201509178299
2. https://www.cancercenter.com/esophageal-cancer/photodynamic-therapy/
3. https://www.cancerquest.org/cancer-biology/cancer-development
4. https://www.ncbi.nlm.nih.gov/pmc/articles/PMC3693758/
5. https://www.ncbi.nlm.nih.gov/pmc/articles/PMC5078657/figure/fig2/
6. http://www.lifeextension.com/Magazine/2016/9/How-Curcumin-Targets-Cancer/Page-01
7. https://www.ncbi.nlm.nih.gov/pubmed/
8. https://www.ncbi.nlm.nih.gov/pubmed/27025786
9. https://www.ncbi.nlm.nih.gov/pubmed/16545122
10. https://www.ncbi.nlm.nih.gov/pubmed/16757216
11. https://www.ncbi.nlm.nih.gov/pubmed/21372035
12. https://www.ncbi.nlm.nih.gov/pubmed/23745991

13. https://www.ncbi.nlm.nih.gov/pubmed/22473809
14. https://www.ncbi.nlm.nih.gov/pubmed/19901561
15. https://www.ncbi.nlm.nih.gov/pubmed/21058202
16. https://www.ncbi.nlm.nih.gov/pubmed/18628464
17. https://www.ncbi.nlm.nih.gov/pubmed/17436567

Chapter 43:

Weight Loss

I am working out every day, but I am not loosing weight. What should I do?

A new international study has shown that food intake can achieve 91% to 93% of weight loss; but exercise can only achieve 7% to 9% of weight loss (1). It is not possible to get on top of a weight problem by exercising only. The better approach to weight loss would be going for a brisk walk and otherwise take care of the nutritional aspect. Calorie restriction is still the most effective way to lose weight.

Having said that, analyze your food intake. I suggest that you write down everything that goes into your mouth for 1 week. I did this with patients when I was in general practice. Then I saw them one week later and I took a red pen encircling everything that made them fat: unnecessary refined carbs; like pasta, white rice, bread, muffins etc. I pointed out the hidden sugar in soft drinks, in cakes, power bars and other processed food.

I asked them to cut out these things I had circled and to come back and see me in another week. I weighed them on each occasion that I saw them and they did lose weight as they made changes. But very few managed to keep it up on the long term, because they slipped back into the old food habits. You need a good dose of motivation and willpower to maintain your newly achieved lower weight. I do it by having permanently cut out sugar and honey. I also permanently stay away from wheat and flour. I replaced pasta, bread, white rice and other starchy foods by vegetables, fruit and salads. It can be done!

One useful tool is a body composition scale that keep track of your body mass index, fat percentage and muscle percentage.

Remember, three tools are necessary to control your eating habits:

1. A piece of paper and pen to record everything you eat.
2. Body composition scales.
3. The third tool is invisible: Willpower!

Internet reference

1. http://www.weightymatters.ca/2016/02/constrained-energy-expenditures-and-not.html

I lost weight on a diet, but now I am afraid of regaining weight, if I eat normally. Can you tell me what to do?

The simplest way is to do what I do. I bought myself body composition scales. They help you to compute your weight, your fat percentage and visceral fat percentage, your muscle percentage and your body mass index. If you weigh yourself daily and record all of these values in a little booklet behind the date, you cannot go wrong. There are small daily fluctuations, but if you eat just the right amount of calories, your values will stay the same. There are publications that say that your best life expectancy is when your body mass index remains within the 21.0 to 22.0 range. This is where I keep my weight.

Keep in mind that our weight depends to 91% to 93% on what we eat and only to 7% to 9% on how much we exercise. This has been measured by a recent study (see link below). Make sure you get balanced meals with protein (dairy products, lean meat, fish), carbs from vegetables and fruit and some fat. You can have nuts and dark chocolate (85%). Current teaching is that 20% of your total daily calories can come from fat. The most important value is your body mass index. With this method you will keep your weight down. I have done it since 2001; I had lost 50 pounds and my BMI has remained at 21.5.

Here is the reference regarding diet counting 91% to 93% of weight loss:

Internet reference

1. http://www.weightymatters.ca/2016/02/constrained-energy-expenditures-and-not.html

How can I get rid of belly fat, and then maintain a good-looking body?

What you are describing is a common problem. It is usually associated with the Standard American diet. You get a burger with French fries when you are hungry, you eat a muffin with a Latte at Starbucks in between meals and you swallow a good-sized steak for dinner with potatoes and bread and butter. Now you feel you also deserve a couple of beers. You call the belly that you have the "beer belly", and it is bad for your health.

Here is the solution of what to do get rid of the beer belly.

1. Remove sugar and high fructose corn syrup from your diet.

2. The second effective step is to cut out as many empty starches that you can cut out like white rice, bread, sweets, cookies, cakes, ice cream and pasta. The reason for this is that these starchy foods get metabolized in the gut into sugar, which causes an insulin response. The extra insulin is responsible for developing inflammation in the arteries, which eventually leads to heart attacks and strokes.

3. Exercise on a regular basis. This will produce HDL cholesterol, the protective cholesterol, which balances LDL cholesterol. I suggest 30 minutes of treadmill followed by 10 weight machines. In the beginning go slow, but gradually increase the incline on the treadmill and the speed; also gradually increase the weights. If you are unsure of what to do, talk to a trainer.

4. Perhaps the most important step is to rebalance your food intake. With this I mean that you replace high glycemic-index carbs with low glycemic-index carbs. This means you will eat a lot of salads, steamed vegetables, and fruit. This gives you a lot of extra fiber, which your system needs to slow down the rate of sugar absorption, helps you to lower LDL cholesterol and helps you to detoxify your body in the gut where toxins are bound to fiber.

5. If you are heavily into alcoholic drinks, you should know that this is another source of refined carbohydrates that gets metabolized into LDL cholesterol, triglycerides and can cause fatty liver disease and liver cirrhosis. A moderate consumption of alcohol (one drink for women per day and two drinks for men per day) lowers the risk of heart attacks and strokes, while excessive alcohol intake increases the risk (1).

6. Bioidentical hormone replacement may be something you have not heard about. But if you are a woman above

the age of 40 or a man above the age of 50 chances are that your natural hormone production from your testicles or adrenal glands (in a man) or from the ovaries or adrenal glands (in a woman) are no longer keeping up with the demand of regular life. Part of the aging process is that is that the production of our sex hormones slows down shortly before menopause in women and shortly before andropause in men. This will not only manifest itself in hot flashes and sleep disturbance in women or in erectile dysfunction and grumpiness in men; it will eventually lead to a lack of energy metabolism in the heart, the brain and other organ systems that have sex hormone receptors. A lack of hormones translates into yet another cause of heart attacks, strokes and certain cancers. This is an area where conventional medicine disagrees with anti-aging medicine. But it is my experience from years in general practice that heart attacks, strokes, colorectal cancer and pancreatic cancer in both sexes, cancer of the breasts, uterus and ovaries in women and prostate cancer in men are indeed more common when natural hormone production has declined.

Here is more info about the beer belly (2).

Internet references

1. http://www.livestrong.com/article/269045-does-alcohol-raise-cholesterol-levels/
2. http://www.askdrray.com/beer-belly-bad-news/

My stomach is outgrowing my pants. Would 30 minutes jogging a day help?

1. Physically this would be good for your cardiovascular system, preventing strokes and heart attacks.

2. But you are thinking about weight loss. There has been a publication that figured that all out. Only 7% to 9% of calorie loss occurs from exercise while dieting provides 91% to 93% of calorie loss. This makes weight loss more effective by dieting:

3. The bottom line: you need to look at what you are eating and modify that. I suspect too much sugar, too many refined carbs as bread, chips, pasta and potatoes. Eat more veggies, salads; have some nuts. Reduce your calorie intake in order to tame that belly! And here is another observation: it took a while for that belly to outgrow your pants. It will also take you some time to lose the weight. Be persistent and patient.

Internet reference

1. http://www.weightymatters.ca/2016/02/constrained-energy-expenditures-and-not.html

How can I lose weight without too much exercise?

You are in luck that you don't have to worry about an extensive exercising program that much. A publication has established that only about 8% of weight loss is due to exercising. 92% of weight loss is due to dieting: "Constrained Energy Expenditures and Not Outrunning Our Forks" (1).

The key to proper dieting is to cut out sugar, processed foods (which also contain loads of sugar) and refined carbs. Research the glycemic index and glycemic load. Then follow the low glycemic index/low glycemic load foods that you will find with your research. I have done this in 2001 and lost 50 pounds. I kept it off by staying on this diet.

Under the chapter "diet" I answered this question: I want to get rid of sugar in my diet. How can I do this long-term? In it I explain what diet I followed to achieve what you would like to do. But for your well being and fitness make daily exercise part of your life: walk a block or more, take the stairs instead of the elevator, walk a longer distance in a parking lot or hit the gym.

Internet reference

1. http://www.weightymatters.ca/2016/02/constrained-energy-expenditures-and-not.html

Can I get a flat belly by just running every day without crunches?

Here we go again. Another question about trying to lose weight by running. It will not work whether you run or do crunches. Weight loss can only be achieved by a proper calorie-poor diet. A proper diet is responsible for weight loss in 92% of cases, exercise only in 8% (1).
More info: How can I lose weight without too much exercise?

Internet reference

1. http://www.weightymatters.ca/2016/02/constrained-energy-expenditures-and-not.html

How can I get rid of my lower belly fat?

It is not difficult to target lower belly fat. If you have that belly fat and you think you can get rid of it by doing nothing, you are misinformed. Your belly got there on the first place because you ate too much sugar, processed foods containing sugar and starch foods (pasta, bread, muffins, donuts, pizza, potatoes, rice etc.).

The remedy to get rid of your belly fat is very simple. Eat vegetables, salads, nuts, fish, lean clean meats (organic chicken and turkey, grass-fed beef, bison meat) and fruit. Leave out the sugar, processed foods and starchy foods. Within just 3 to 4 months you will lose your entire superfluous belly fat. How do I know? Because I did this in 2001 and have kept it up since. It works!

Chapter 44:

Younger for Longer

Why are some people younger looking than their stated age?

Some of this may be genetic. In Asian countries it is not unusual that people look 10 to 15 years younger than they are. In Indonesians I have also noticed that they often look significantly younger than they are. Whether or not they turn older is a secondary question.

In my opinion stress is a major aging factor, so are lifestyles like drinking too much alcohol and smoking. So, before you engage in any of the recommendations below, work on those obvious aging factors. Stop smoking, cut down alcoholic drinks to a bare minimum (or cut it out altogether) and control stress.

Everybody has access to anti-aging methods:

1. You can take vitamins and minerals in addition to eating a Mediterranean type diet. This can add 9 to 10 years of life, particularly vitamin C and E.

2. You can add bioidentical hormones, which makes you 15 years younger, if you start right away when menopause sets in or andropause in males.

3. Older people should have their blood tested for IGF-1 levels or overnight urine for human growth hormone metabolites. If human growth hormone is low, it can be replaced by an insulin-like needle injection containing pure growth hormone (HGH). A dose of only 0.1 mg to 0.2 mg human growth hormone per night, given daily will add 26.5 years on average, if deficiency of HGH was documented before replacing it. It will flatten out wrinkles, treat joint problems, and preserve muscle mass together with bioidentical sex hormone replacement. This data comes from Dr. Hertoghe, who gave several lectures at the 23rd Annual World Congress on Anti-Aging Medicine on Dec. 13, 2015 in Las Vegas. He is an endocrinologist from Belgium and his talk was entitled "How to extend the human lifespan by 40 years". It was a fascinating lecture (1).

4. Of course you need to keep up your daily exercise that should include 30-minutes of treadmill and 20 to 25 minutes of weight machines.

5. Also keep alcohol in moderation as mentioned above. Remember that alcohol is an aging substance. Often people who consume a lot of alcohol look 10 to 15 years older than they are!

Internet reference

1. http://www.askdrray.com/life-extended-by-several-decades/

When do we develop wrinkles in our face?

Wrinkles develop as a combination of skin damage from sunlight exposure and lack of hormone production as we age, particularly the lack of human growth hormone (HGH).

Dr. Hertoghe, an endocrinologist from Belgium gave a lecture at the 23rd Annual World Congress on Anti-Aging Medicine on Dec. 13, 2015 in Las Vegas that I attended. He talked about the life-prolonging effect of human HGH. He explained that he has done blood tests (IGF-1) and also 24-hour urine metabolite tests of HGH on aging patients and found that many are deficient with regard to HGH production. He explained that from age 35 onwards GH is not released as much as in the past by the pituitary gland and this causes the aging process to get accelerated with wrinkles around the face area. At the same time HGH deficiency, which is much more common than generally acknowledged, is also responsible for aging of the vital organs and of the musculoskeletal system causing disabilities and premature death.

But Dr. Hertoghe also said that this aging process (wrinkles, vital organ aging etc.) is reversible when you inject a tiny amount of human growth hormone daily using an injection pen (like an insulin injector with a tiny needle). The dosage is between 0.1mg to 0.2 mg at bedtime daily and must be monitored by the treating physician. He showed before and after images and I was amazed that wrinkles can actually disappear. This is not something you can do by yourself (except for the injections); you need a doctor who has experience with this. Also, don't expect miracles overnight. It takes between 1 and 3 years for the healing process to take place. Another problem at this point are the expenses, although in some countries a special drug plan will pay for the expenses, as HGH deficiency is a true hormone deficiency like diabetes.

Publications of medical questions and answers in popular magazines.

Ibtimes.com: July 16, 2017

How to Stay Young: 5 Tips To Reverse Aging

Answer by Ray Schilling, M.D., author of "Healing Gone Wrong, Healing Done Right".

   1. Exercise regularly. Those who do exercise regularly have only 50% of the major diseases like heart attacks, strokes, cancer, diabetes and arthritis.
   2. Eat sensibly, meaning eat a balanced diet like the Mediterranean diet. Here is a review of the main benefits of a Mediterranean diet: 8 Health Benefits of the Mediterranean Diet - Dr. Axe (1).
   3. Learn how to relax; use any of the following methods: meditation, self-hypnosis, yoga or Tai Chi. Relaxation Techniques for Health (2).
   4. When you are aging, you will first encounter menopause, if you are a woman or andropause, if you are a man. The key is to measure what hormones are missing and replace the missing hormones with bioidentical hormones (3). But there are other hormones like melatonin, thyroid and human growth hormone that may also be lacking.
   5. Supplement with life-prolonging supplements: vitamin C, vitamin D3, resveratrol, CoQ10, quercetin, omega-3 fatty acids (fish oil). Supplement added to standard diet improves health, prolongs life in mice.

Internet references

1. https://draxe.com/mediterranean-diet/
2. https://nccih.nih.gov/health/stress/relaxation.htm

3. https://www.bodylogicmd.com/bioidentical-hormone-therapy?gclid=Cj0KEQjwv_fKBRCG8a3ao-OQuZ8BEiQAvpH6ld7dXvhXjbbfazksfZrYkvE4k6dqWkqz3Skwl3lRHgaAgYm8P8HAQ&tid=cpc.google.g.out_of_market_geo.bioidentical.%2Bbioidentical+%2Bhormones.b.c.%7Badid%7D.1406756188
4. https://www.sciencedaily.com/releases/2014/02/140227125240.htm

What are three things I can do every day to stay younger for longer?

1. Daily exercise to keep your arteries open and condition your cardiovascular system. It also prevents falls as you get older, because your muscles will sustain you and your balance organs will continue to function well with exercise keeping you from falling.

2. Bioidentical hormone replacement: This is important in a multitude of ways.

• Melatonin is depleted above the age of 20. But taking 3 mg of melatonin at bedtime keeps your immune system healthy, helps you to sleep better and regulates the other hormones.

• An aging male will likely require testosterone replacement (as bioidentical testosterone cream) or as injection twice per week. Keep total testosterone levels in your blood between 500 and 1000 ng/dl. So a goal of 700 to 800 ng/dl would be reasonable.

• Women beyond menopause need progesterone, because there is no longer a corpus luteum in the ovaries without menstruation. They may also require a small amount of estradiol. See a knowledgeable health care provider for bioidentical hormone replacement. This point can make you look and feel 10 to 15 years younger.

• Finally, many people underestimate the power of human growth hormone HGH). An overpowering feeling of exhaustion can be due to HGH deficiency:

Internet reference

https://www.ncbi.nlm.nih.gov/pmc/articles/PMC3183535/

• This is diagnosed by taking insulin-like growth factor-1 (IGF-1) levels. When these are low, daily subcutaneous injection of low-dose human growth hormone is given. Depending on how severe growth hormone deficiency is, different HGH doses are administered. The patient self-injects with an insulin injector. Mild HGH deficiency requires 0.05 mg (1 click) per day, moderate deficiency 0.1 mg (2 clicks) per day and severe deficiency 0.15 mg (3 clicks) per day. See this link: Hormone Changes With Burnout:

Internet reference

http://www.askdrray.com/hormone-changes-with-burnout/

3. A balanced diet without added sugar, avoiding processed foods and cutting out all empty starchy foods will help you to stay younger for longer. The Mediterranean diet comes to mind, but other diets like the Zone diet and the DASH diet are all good alternatives. Whatever you do, avoid the American Standard diet, which would age you prematurely.

Chapter 45:

Summary

I have answered a lot of questions from other people and have shared with you my answers. But now it is time for you to think what questions you would like to ask your treating physician. I have a few suggestions for you.

- Do I have to take this medication for the rest of my life?
- Do I really need this X-ray? Could I get leukemia from that down the road?
- What is the cause of all my symptoms?
- What could I do to prevent this from happening again?

You may not always get satisfying answers to your questions. But sometimes you get initial answers that help you cope for the time being. Then, when circumstances change, you may have more questions and the answers to these may be more meaningful for you. Don't be afraid to ask questions. They are the key to medical solutions concerning your health. If you want to solve your health problems, you must attempt to get an answer to what the cause of your symptoms is. Many health professionals just treat your symptoms, but this will not give you a long-term solution.

There is also the problem of getting side effects from the medicine that was prescribed for you. If there are lifestyle changes you can make, that will treat the cause of your problems, don't procrastinate. Make the changes now! Lifestyle changes have no side effects, while medication often has. All the big diseases like diabetes, heart disease and arthritis respond to a certain extent to lifestyle changes. Healthy nutrition and regular exercise are two powerful recipes for health. "Medical Questions Answered" has attempted to answer specific health questions. I will continue to answer questions regarding longevity in this blog (1). Answers to questions about various general health concerns can be found on this blog (2).

I hope that you engage in healthy lifestyle practices and continue to look for answers regarding your own health problems.

Internet references

1. http://www.askdrray.com/
2. http://nethealthbook.com/news

Index

A

Acne 1-7

AGEs (Advanced glycation end products) 258

Aging xxi, 9-17, 20, 22-24, 26, 28, 35, 38, 40, 49, 60, 74, 83, 86, 90, 91, 101, 171, 186, 188, 189, 191, 204, 206, 207, 208-213, 215, 219, 223, 226, 240, 241, 258, 264, 265, 269, 270, 287, 291, 292-295

Alcohol 2, 14, 23, 31, 32, 35, 51, 58, 81, 97, 132, 173, 180, 195, 208, 223, 224, 240, 241, 246, 286, 291, 292

Alzheimer's disease xxi, 14, 18, 24, 33-44, 74, 90, 93, 114, 130, 131, 155, 166, 169, 172, 177, 203, 204, 205, 208, 220, 223, 258, 259, 265, 266, 267

Androgens 4, 185, 187

Andropause 11, 26, 40, 49, 82, 83, 183-185, 194, 226, 248, 287, 292, 294

Anti-aging medicine 15, 21, 23, 28, 207, 212, 219, 240, 241, 287, 292, 293

Appearance 12, 13, 46, 58, 202

Arachidonic acid 19

Arthritis xxi, 19, 42, 47-49, 55, 111, 114, 118, 131, 132, 138, 139, 154, 176, 208, 226, 258, 265, 266, 267, 294, 298

Autism 53, 54, 235, 261, 267

B

Back pain xxi, 28, 55-57

Barrier methods 89

Beans 37, 108, 141, 204

Bioflavonoids 120, 266

Bioidentical hormone replacement 15, 40, 49, 82, 83, 185, 187, 189, 201, 207, 209, 212, 226, 248, 286, 295

BMI (body mass index) 107, 173, 285

Bone 5, 14, 18, 20, 23, 27, 49, 84, 90, 157, 164, 165, 168, 186, 192, 211, 221, 226, 231, 232, 236, 263, 264, 268, 272

Bone marrow failure 14, 27, 90

Bovine growth hormone 136

Brain 6, 14, 18, 23, 24, 27, 31, 33-39, 41-44, 58, 90, 92-94, 97, 98, 100-102, 112, 114, 117, 131, 149, 150, 154, 162, 166, 168, 170, 172, 175, 177, 186,

187, 202, 203, 204, 211, 235, 237, 244, 249, 251, 264, 287

Brain cancer 6, 149

Brain health 36, 38, 203, 205

Breast cancer 60, 61, 77, 87, 124, 125, 126, 127, 128, 190-193, 221, 279, 280

C

Calories 16, 104, 105, 106, 121, 129, 173, 174, 180, 265, 285

Cancer xvii, xviii, xxi, xxii, 6, 7, 14, 19, 20, 23, 27, 29-31, 38, 42, 51, 60-87, 90, 93, 114, 123-128, 130, 133, 141-144, 149, 155, 168, 187-193, 204, 208, 212, 216, 217, 220, 221, 223, 224, 231-235, 254, 258, 259, 266, 267, 273-281, 287, 294

Cancer cure xxi, 64, 75, 234, 274

Cancer research xvii, 64, 65, 84, 216-218, 275, 276

Carb diet 115, 126, 128, 172, 259

Carbohydrates 36, 106, 108, 109, 112, 116, 127, 129, 174, 286

Carcinogens 60, 61, 62, 63, 78, 80, 81, 142, 176, 192, 274

Cardiovascular disease 83, 90, 165, 166, 167, 169, 208, 257, 266

Cause of cancer 128, 258

Cereals 37, 113, 144, 204

Cervical cancer 221, 234, 276

Cheese 106, 107, 108, 136, 173, 260

Chelation treatment 24, 54, 262

Cholesterol 18, 19, 36, 42, 111-115, 120-123, 134, 164, 166, 167, 169-177, 219, 257, 260, 264, 266, 286

Colon cancer 77, 124, 142, 155, 216, 278

Constipation 141-145

Contraception 88, 89

Conventional medicine 55, 56, 192, 227, 287

Co-Q 10 16, 264, 265

Corn syrup 131, 286

Coronary arteries 24, 152, 154, 165, 166, 173, 221

C-reactive protein 166, 170, 171

Cryotherapy 29, 72, 73, 76-79, 86

Cryoablation therapy 64, 275

D

DASH diet 38, 42, 43, 105, 167, 175, 180, 204, 223, 296

Death 13, 14, 31, 69, 75, 90, 91, 121, 171, 172, 181, 182, 197, 202, 220, 221, 222, 251, 254, 257, 274, 293

Dementia 20, 27, 33, 35, 36, 40, 41, 43, 166, 172, 203, 208, 241, 267

Depression 6, 35, 57, 92-98, 100-102, 143, 186, 235, 243, 267

Detoxification 24, 68, 103, 146

Diabetes 33-35, 38, 40, 42, 94, 101, 104, 105, 118, 124, 127, 130, 131, 166, 172, 173, 177, 180, 205, 208, 223, 235, 236, 257-259, 265-269, 293, 294, 298

Diet xxi, 1-3, 5, 6, 9, 14, 19, 23, 26, 36, 37-39, 42-44, 47, 50, 51, 61, 63, 79, 81, 97, 104-106, 109, 111, 113-117, 124, 126-128, 130-133, 143, 144, 153, 165-167, 169, 172, 173, 175, 177, 180, 182, 190, 203-206, 208, 210, 218, 222, 223, 226, 257-260, 274, 284-286, 288, 289, 291, 294, 296

Dietary approach 6, 104

Digestion 105, 129, 138

Discectomy 55

Disease xxi, xxii, 13, 14, 18, 19, 22, 24, 31-42, 47, 51, 52, 55, 60, 63, 69, 70, 74, 77-80, 83, 90, 93-97, 105, 111, 114, 124, 130-132, 136, 144, 159, 160, 163, 164-169, 172, 173, 177, 178, 185, 197, 203-205, 207, 208, 214, 220, 221, 223, 224, 235, 236, 257-259, 264-269, 277, 279, 280, 286, 294, 298

Diurnal rhythm 241, 250, 253

DNA 9, 10, 16, 17, 22, 25, 27, 60, 64, 74, 90, 91, 206, 210, 212, 213, 236, 265, 268, 269, 274

Doctor 10, 11, 28, 29, 44, 50, 82, 89, 139, 140, 143, 148, 149, 150, 160, 169, 170, 172, 179, 184, 187, 188, 191, 193, 194, 195, 207, 211, 223, 227, 232, 255, 293

E

Early cancer detection xxii, 217

Esophageal cancer 61, 64, 275

Exercise xxi, 9, 10, 16, 17, 23, 26, 29, 35, 37-41, 44, 48, 50, 63, 75, 80, 81, 83, 92, 98, 107,

130, 152-154, 157, 164-169, 171, 171, 174, 177, 186, 190, 204-206, 211, 220, 222, 223, 226, 253, 264, 265, 274, 283, 285, 286, 288, 289, 292, 294, 295, 298

Exercising regularly 15, 214

F

Fat 14, 19, 37, 101, 105-108, 110, 113-117, 121, 127, 132-134, 144, 147, 168, 172-174, 177, 185, 190, 204, 258-260, 283-286, 289, 290

FDA 74, 82, 96, 177, 182, 191, 258, 259, 279

Fish 2, 37, 105, 106, 107, 108, 119, 132, 176, 203, 204, 285

Fish oil 80, 81, 97, 132, 176, 206, 267, 294

Foot problems 157

Fruit 2, 37, 108, 109, 111, 113, 117, 119, 120, 122, 144, 146, 169, 174, 175, 204, 206, 258, 266, 284, 285, 286, 290

Fusion surgery 56

G

Glucose 64, 67, 104, 105, 112, 119, 236, 268, 275

Gluten 94, 120-122, 159, 160

Gluten free 120-122, 159

Gout 51, 52, 132

Green tea 75, 81, 82, 208, 266, 269

Growth hormone deficiency 10, 209, 211, 296

Gut disease 159

H

Hardening of arteries 112, 121, 258

HDL cholesterol 18, 114, 134, 164, 166, 173, 175, 219, 286

Healthy lifestyles 9, 210

Heart xxi, 10, 13, 14, 18, 19, 20, 23, 24, 27, 31, 32, 35, 38, 39, 42, 62, 63, 74, 83, 90, 111, 112, 114, 118, 120-123, 130-132, 150-154, 162-178, 181, 182, 185-191, 201, 204, 205, 211, 219, 221-224, 236, 254, 257-260, 263-269, 286, 287, 294, 298

Heart attack 10, 13, 18-20, 24, 32, 35, 38, 39, 42, 62, 63, 74, 83, 90, 111, 112, 114, 118, 120-123, 130, 131, 150-152, 154, 164, 166-168, 170-177, 187-191, 204, 205, 211, 219, 221, 223, 224, 236, 254, 257-260, 263-268, 286, 287, 294

Heart disease xxi, 18, 63, 111, 132, 164, 165, 173, 177, 178, 185, 221, 264, 266, 267, 269, 298

Heart failure 14, 24, 27, 31, 90, 182, 264

Heavy metals 24, 35, 54, 262

Hemoglobin A1C 173

HGH (human growth hormone) 10, 12, 22, 26, 28, 29, 48, 49, 117, 136, 189, 207, 209, 211, 223, 226, 240, 243, 248-251, 253, 292-296

HGH metabolite test 29, 49, 226

High blood pressure 14, 16, 19, 38, 55, 112, 118, 131, 167, 179, 180-182, 204, 236, 266, 268

Hip replacement 14

Hippocampus 34, 35, 37, 40, 43, 203

Hormones 3, 4, 10-13, 15, 20, 22, 24, 26, 40, 41, 48, 49, 82, 83, 100-102, 116, 117, 169, 183, 185-191, 193, 194, 201, 207, 212, 223, 226, 235, 239-242, 244, 246, 247, 248, 250, 251, 253, 254, 256, 287, 292, 294, 295

Hormone deficiencies 11, 28, 48, 49, 193, 211, 226, 239

Hormone replacement 15, 28, 29, 40, 49, 82, 83, 94, 184, 185, 187, 188, 189, 194, 201, 207, 209, 212, 226, 248, 286, 292, 295

Hospital xvii, 30, 96, 127, 148, 183, 184, 195, 202, 217

H. pylori 138, 139, 140

Hypertension 179, 180, 181, 182

Hypoglycemia 118

I

IBS (irritable bowel syndrome) 159, 160,

IGF (insulin growth factor) 1, 2, 4-7, 10, 12, 22, 29, 8, 49, 209, 211, 226, 248, 292, 293, 296

Immune response xvii

Immunotherapy 66, 78, 79, 84

Indole-3-carbinol 190

Infections 14, 81, 197, 221

Infertility 208, 236, 268

Inflammation 18, 19, 35, 42, 80, 81, 83, 94, 97, 98, 111, 114, 118, 130, 131, 132, 134, 161, 166, 169, 171, 177, 198, 206, 223, 258, 265-267, 269, 276, 286

Injections of HGH 49

Injuries xviii, 56, 200

Insulin 4, 5, 7, 10, 12, 18, 22, 34, 35, 40, 42, 43, 49, 63, 94, 97, 98, 101, 105, 109, 112, 114, 118-121, 124, 126-128,

130, 133, 166, 173, 209, 211, 226, 248, 260, 266, 269, 274, 286, 292, 293, 296

Insulin resistance 94, 97, 101, 105, 124, 126, 127, 128, 133, 173, 266, 269

Integrative medicine 50, 55, 99, 227

K

Kidney failure 14, 27, 90, 143, 170

L

LDL cholesterol 18, 36, 42, 111, 112, 113, 114, 115, 120, 121-123, 134, 164, 166, 167, 169, 171, 173, 174, 176, 177, 219, 257, 258, 260, 264, 266, 286

Leaky gut syndrome 118, 160, 214

Lean meat 105, 106, 285, 290

Leukemia 14, 51, 84, 85, 221, 297

Life expectancy 12, 17, 22, 23, 25, 28, 60, 61, 80, 152, 206, 209, 210, 212, 220 222, 244, 258, 259, 263, 269, 285

Lifestyle 9, 16, 23, 35, 38, 40, 41, 165, 168, 173, 177, 181, 187, 207, 210, 214, 265, 291, 298

Lifestyle changes 16, 23, 181, 265, 298

Liver cancer 14, 81, 124, 187, 188, 224

Liver cirrhosis 14, 31, 81, 224, 286

Liver failure 14, 27, 31

Low carb diet 126, 128

Low-glycemic diet 1, 6, 257

Low-glycemic index 1, 6, 128

Lung cancer 62, 64, 80, 221, 223

M

Medical questions xvii, xviii, xxi, 13, 65, 80, 100, 112, 200, 207, 214, 225, 252, 294, 298

Meditation 9, 26, 83, 208, 210, 220, 223, 294

Mediterranean diet 9, 15, 23, 26, 36-39, 42, 43, 44, 50, 81, 83, 97, 105, 113, 115-117, 133, 166, 169, 172, 203-206, 208, 210, 222, 226, 259, 274, 294, 296

Melatonin 11-13, 26, 40, 83, 116, 117, 189, 194, 223, 239-244, 246-255, 266, 269, 294, 295

Memory loss 34-36, 40

Menopause 11, 20, 26, 40, 49, 82, 83, 168, 183, 188, 194,

208, 222, 226, 248, 287, 292, 294, 295

Mercury 24, 53, 132, 176, 261

Metabolism 15, 16,19, 26, 40, 53, 63, 64, 67, 112-114, 123, 124, 126, 166, 167, 172, 174, 212, 236, 261, 265, 268, 272, 274, 287

Metal processing metabolism 53, 261

Methylation defect 167, 235, 267, 270

Migraines 191, 235, 268

Milk products 1, 5, 7, 136

MIND diet 38, 42, 43, 44, 204

Mitochondria 9, 10, 15-17, 20, 22, 25, 26, 27, 64, 90, 91,112,162,174, 206, 210, 211, 213, 258, 264, 265, 269, 275

My background xvii, xviii

N

NSAIDs (non-steroidal anti-inflammatory drugs) 138, 139, 225

Nutrition 1, 10, 35, 108, 110, 115, 116, 131, 162, 165, 208, 211, 253, 283, 298

Nuts 12, 37, 109, 117, 132, 172, 173, 204, 247, 251, 260, 285, 288, 290

O

Obesity 35, 43, 115, 124, 131, 165, 166, 180, 183, 184, 208, 259

Old age 12, 13, 14, 24, 40, 60, 74, 90, 91

Olive oil 19, 20, 23, 37, 106, 109, 114, 166, 169, 172, 173, 204

Omega-3 fatty acid 2, 9, 19, 20, 50, 97, 114, 132, 176, 180, 192, 193, 208, 210, 227, 267, 294

Omega-6 fatty acid 19,132

Osteoarthritis 49, 154, 226, 265, 266

Osteoporosis 14,18, 20, 23, 165, 168, 169, 208, 222, 258, 263, 264, 267, 272

P

P53 gene 64, 274

Pain xxi, 5, 11, 24, 26, 28, 48, 49, 50, 55-57, 132, 134, 142, 143, 148, 150, 157, 158, 171, 177, 193, 198-200, 225, 226, 236, 268

Pain relief 225

Pancreatic cancer 6, 31, 61, 124, 127, 221, 224, 279, 280, 287

Parenting 228

Parkinson's disease 42, 93, 131, 208

Phototherapy 64, 235, 268, 275

Photodynamic laser therapy 66, 73

Physical activity 9, 98, 143, 174, 208, 210, 214

Pimples 1, 3, 4, 6

Pineal gland 11, 116, 189, 194-241, 246, 249, 253, 266

Plantar fasciitis 157, 158

Platelet-rich plasma 49, 226

Pneumonia xviii, 146, 199, 221

Polycystic ovary syndrome 4

Popularity of questions xxi

Postmenopausal women 18, 20, 172, 263

Poultry 37, 106, 204

PQQ (Pyrroloquinoline quinone) 16, 22, 264, 265

Pregnancy 88, 89, 229, 230

Premature aging 12, 20, 186, 258

Proactive xxii

Probiotics 61, 118

Processed foods 3, 19, 42, 81, 113, 118, 119, 121, 132, 133, 134, 258, 259, 288, 290, 296

Prolong life 23, 152, 269, 270

Prolotherapy 49, 55, 56, 226

Prostate cancer 20, 29, 61, 64, 66, 70, 72, 73, 76, 77, 78, 85, 86, 87, 189, 190, 231, 232, 233, 234, 275, 280, 287

Protein 4, 5, 73, 76, 116, 124, 133, 166, 170, 174, 177, 258, 285

Q

Quinoa 160

Quit smoking 206, 222

R

Red meat 61, 132

Regular sex life 11, 28, 193, 194

Relaxation 9, 57, 83, 186, 206, 208, 210, 220, 223, 294

Resveratrol 9, 16, 18, 81, 175, 208, 210, 264, 265, 266, 294

Rheumatoid arthritis 47, 48, 55, 265

S

SAD diet (Standard American diet) 23, 42, 131, 285, 296

Salads 20, 105, 227, 284, 286, 288, 290

Schizophrenia 235, 267, 196

Sebaceous gland 4, 5

Serotonin 34, 35, 92, 95, 97, 100, 101, 252

Sex life 11, 28, 29, 193, 194

Skin 4, 5, 20, 29, 32, 46, 68, 77, 82, 103, 201, 202, 209, 238, 272, 276, 292

Skin cancer 77, 276

Sleep xxi, 11, 12, 27, 34-36, 40, 116, 117, 118, 168, 193, 194, 198, 206, 208, 218, 225, 239-256, 266, 287, 295

Sleep deprivation 36, 252

Sleep pattern xxi, 117, 248

Sleep problems 11, 194, 239

Smoking 23, 60-63, 80, 180, 206, 208, 220-223, 224, 291, 35, 39

SPECT scans 58

Sperm 16, 88, 89, 213, 230

Starchy foods 18, 97, 106, 113, 114, 116, 117, 127, 128, 130, 131, 134, 164, 166, 214, 257, 260, 284, 286, 290, 296

Statins 170, 171, 172, 174, 177

Stem cell therapy 49, 55, 56, 212, 226

Stomach cancer 61, 221

Stress 4, 12, 19, 35, 40, 44, 48, 57, 83, 114, 116, 139, 154, 157, 168, 175, 206, 208, 219, 220, 225, 239, 241, 242, 247, 249, 253, 254, 269, 291

Strokes 10, 13, 14, 18-20, 32, 38, 39, 42, 62, 63, 74, 83, 90, 93, 111, 112, 114, 118, 120-123, 130-132, 152, 154, 164, 166-168, 170-177, 185, 187, 189-191, 198, 205, 211, 219, 223, 224, 254, 257-260, 263-267, 286, 287, 294

Sugar 1-4, 7, 18, 19, 33, 34, 36, 40, 42, 43, 63, 67, 80, 81, 94, 97, 101, 106-123, 124-128, 129-131, 133-135, 145, 164, 166, 169, 173, 180, 206, 214, 246, 257-260, 264, 274, 283, 284, 286-290, 296

Suicide 93, 96, 98, 270

Supplements 16, 20, 22-24, 26, 41, 50, 80, 81, 83, 98, 167, 169, 171, 174, 176, 177, 206, 211, 227, 237, 263-265, 267, 269, 270, 273, 294

Sweetener 36, 109, 111, 119, 120, 121, 135

T

Teenagers 1-5

Telomeres 9, 10, 12, 25, 26, 27, 38, 204, 207-210, 213, 223, 225, 242, 250, 254, 263

Testosterone 4, 9, 11-13, 20, 26, 28, 29, 48, 49, 82, 101, 168, 183-190, 192-194, 208, 210, 226, 239, 240, 246-248, 250, 253, 295

Thyroid-stimulating hormone 11, 192

Total hip replacement 49, 154, 226

Total knee replacement 49, 154, 226

Tryptophan 93, 94, 100, 101

TSH (thyroid stimulating hormone) 11, 28, 102, 192, 193

Type-3 diabetes 33, 40, 166

U

Ulcers 55, 138, 139, 140

V

Vaccinations 53, 261

Vegetables 2, 37, 81, 105, 108, 109, 113, 117, 120, 130, 142, 144, 160, 167, 174, 175, 180, 190, 204, 206, 226, 260, 266, 284-286, 290

Vitamins 62, 109, 115, 164, 169, 177, 206, 208, 209, 235, 263, 265, 267, 269, 270, 291

Vitamin A 5

Vitamin B 93, 98, 100, 167, 169, 177, 235, 236, 268

Vitamin C 9, 81, 109, 208, 210, 269, 291, 294

Vitamin D3 9, 15, 23, 26, 41, 44, 50, 80, 81, 97, 164-169, 206, 208, 210, 227, 264, 266, 269, 272, 273, 294

Vitamin E 9, 175, 208, 269

Vitamin K2 18, 23, 164, 167, 169, 263, 272

W

Weight 17, 18, 37, 39, 104, 105, 106, 107, 111, 114, 116-118, 127, 129, 130, 153, 164-166, 173, 179, 182, 190, 204, 222, 257, 283-286, 288, 289, 292

Weight loss 39, 104, 129, 130, 153, 173, 179, 182, 190, 283, 285, 288, 289

Western style diet 1

Wheat 2, 3, 4, 7, 47, 118, 130, 131, 159, 160, 180, 214, 284

Wrinkles 12, 68, 169, 208, 241, 292, 293

Y

Yoga 9, 26, 83, 208, 210, 220, 223, 294

Younger for longer 23, 291, 295, 296

Youth 24

Z

Zinc 206, 236, 268

Made in the USA
Las Vegas, NV
03 April 2024

88211753R00184